PHILOSOPHY AND FAITH OF SIKHISM

PHILOSOPHY AND FAITH OF SIKHISM

by K.S. Duggal

Love Offering by Sri Swami Rama

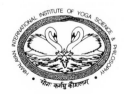

The Himalayan International Institute
of Yoga Science and Philosophy of the U.S.A.
Honesdale, Pennsylvania

Contents

To Rammi and Shehla

*The Paths may be two
but the goal is the same.*

Guru Nanak

A Love Offering

The Sikh philosophy is explained in part by the very word used to identify the Divine—*Waheguru*—the wondrous, wonderful God. *Wahe* means "awesome"; the word *guru* in the true sense means "that which dispels the darkness of ignorance." *Waheguru* is the word or name of the Divine, that which is beyond body, senses, breath, and mind. This is the center of the Sikh spiritual practice. *Waheguru*—the Divine—is the only One, Absolute, Ultimate Reality.

The Sikh philosophy, discipline, and approach is called *Sahaja*, the Easy Way. Its core tenets and beliefs belong to all time and are universal. They are focused on a practical sadhana and reject abstract philosophizing, which is thought only to increase the ego and create barriers for the aspirant.

Thus, the faith and philosophy of Sikh dharma are closely related—in fact, intermingled—in keeping with the Sikh emphasis on a philosophy that has direct implications for one's daily life. For Sikhs, the main purpose of life is the realization of the Lord of Creation, which can only be accomplished through the twin forces of love and the grace of the true guru. The first duty of the disciple is the remembrance of the name of the Lord, the only sacred karma.

In responding to their time, the Sikh gurus created a new order. Their philosophy was not that of the past—that the world was a deluding snare or trap that should be rejected through asceticism, renunciation, or mere philosophical inquiry. Rather, the Sikh philosophy describes the world as a means and a context for human spiritual life. This philosophy rejects renunciation and the path of the ascetic monks, who abandoned their duties and responsibilities, smeared their bodies with ashes, and left the cities to wander in the woods, villages, and on riverbanks with their begging bowls, doing mortifications. The Sikh gurus were consistently critical of these wandering beggars who cut themselves off from their culture and became parasites, never contributing to the welfare of their nation and fellow men.

They were equally critical of those who engaged in external rituals and rites for public show or formalism. They declined to believe that the seeker needed the intervention of priestly wisdom to obtain the divine experience. The Sikh message also abandoned the narrow philosophical and mere intellectual approach, believing that the intellectual gymnasium only increases the disruptive effect of egoism *(Haumey)*, rather than bringing about *Hukum* (a will surrendered to God).

The gurus abandoned the single-minded paths of Bhakti and Karma as they had previously been narrowly practiced, seeing instead a need for a philosophical approach that combined and transcended all these spiritual paths of *Jnana, Bhakti,* and *Karma.*

In this path, the most important practice was the constant assimilation of the Lord's name, so that it becomes a prominent habit of the human mind and heart, and it becomes the leading habit during the time of final transition. The day of departure then becomes a preparation for the spiritual wedding of the soul with the Divine, which is a festive occasion. No mourning, no grief, and no sorrow are necessary, for parting becomes meeting with the Beloved. Death for intellectuals still today is a mystery, but when one prepares himself or herself for the voyage from known to unknown, that preparation is filled with ecstasy, and actually it is not a parting moment but a joyous meeting. The practice of remembering the Lord's name is carried out while the seeker also maintains an actively balanced life in the world.

Philosophically as well, the Sikh gurus rejected the notion of pessimism, passivity, and ritualism, in which the common man felt dependent on the rituals and priestly wisdom to intervene with the divine. The Sikh philosophy is one of humanism—that if the Lord is omnipresent, he is immanent in all. It teaches that a kind of Bhakti or love emphasizing devotion to some aspect of the Divine is only useful if it also realizes that the Divine exists in the hearts of other human beings.

During the time of Nanak Dev, the wave of renunciation was prevalent. Nanak Dev, like Kabir, established that marriage is a holy act and that renunciation is not the only path to salvation. Leading the householder's life while following dharma is equally helpful to the aspirant. Today, the modern psychologists talk much about humanism, and I want to motivate modern psychologists to dive into the sayings of the *Granth Sahib*, in which they will find all the humanistic principles laid down 500 years ago by Sri Nanak Dev, a prophet, seer, and guide of humanity.

This aspect of Sikhism should be explored and used by the modern psychologists and I am hopeful that my next book will be on the subject of the psychology of Sikhism, in which we are going to explore the themes which are most useful for modern man in order to weave a new fabric of understanding for approaching the ailments of stress faced by the modern man.

Guru Nanak Dev created a bridge between two great cultures, religions, and traditions. He changed his society by his simple sayings, which are found in *Granth Sahib*, one of the finest and simplest bibles of the world.

The Sikh Gurus experienced that all aspirants were equal in the sight of the guru, and they utterly rejected both the caste system and the notion of women as an evil or worldly force that intervened in spirituality. All the Sikh gurus expressed this philosophical approach practically—all were married and maintained families and relationships in their community. Further, their philosophy of humanism took the form of believing that love for fellowmen—to be expressed in good works—was a path to opening the heart to love of the Divine. The Sikh gurus built homes, irrigation systems, schools, and public kitchens to provide direct support and practical assistance to their congregations.

The Sikh philosophy of a practical life in the world, which is also aimed at achieving the Divine, was expressed by all the Sikh gurus, who were thought of as the physical manifestations of the primal guru, the Lord himself. Nanak Dev, the founder of Sikhism, was realistic in his approach and his footprints were followed, and his voice was echoed, by the nine gurus who succeeded him. All of them added something to the *Panth*—the path which is called Sikhism—and thus, the glorious path became known and embraced by the poor and rich, equally. Following Guru Gobind Singh, the last of the Sikh gurus, the force of the guru was thought to be manifested in the *Sri Adi Granth,* the extensive holy book compiled by the gurus, which offers universal teachings. Grace is also brought about through the force of *satsanga*, participation in the community life. To the Sikhs, there is no distinction between love of fellow man and love of God.

The Sikh gurus merged the philosophical ideals of the *jnani*, the knower of the *Granth Sahib,* with the *gurmukh,* one who was anointed, the ideal man of truth, who lives in the world like a lotus, yet remains unaffected. The goal is ecstasy and emancipation in this life. The seeker should have no personal, selfish goals except that of becoming worthy of the Lord's love.

Spiritual Practice

The primary spiritual practice of the Sikhs was called *sahaj bhava,* meditating in spontaneity on God's name in the heart. This practice does not preclude one's daily activities of work and care for others. Thus, the Sikh gurus created no practices that involved suppression of basic human needs and instincts, in accordance with an emphasis on non-violence to oneself. They also taught the active cultivation of love toward others, through right thought, action, and speech to purify the ego. Prior to the Sikh gurus, earthly love was seen as a force of *moha* (ignorance), which was an earthly bond only to be broken. In contrast, the Sikh gurus' practice was aimed at elevating the love of the seeker so that it could lead to consciousness of the Lord's glory. They did not allow their love to become abstract or removed from the world because they did not see such love as the capacity of saints alone, but of even the common man or woman.

In fact, one of the core metaphors used by the Sikh gurus in describing the spiritual path was the identification of the seeker with the feminine aspect, the bride, who constantly longs for her bridegroom, the Lord. The goal of the seeker is to create and intensify this longing for the Divine, through all the activities of one's daily life.

The spiritual essence of Sikhism is:

Ek	Absolute Spirit (the One)
Oamkar	Protector/Lord Supreme
Sat(i)	Reality, Eternal (Real)
Naam(u)	Manifest in Truth
Kartaa	Principle of Creation
Purakh(u)	Divine Person
Nirbhau	Controlled by None
Nirvair(u)	Contradicted by None
Akaal	Reality Transcending Time
Moorat(i)	Immanent in Cosmic Form
Ajooni	Not Cast in the Womb
Saibham	Self-Installed
Gur	Enlightener of All
Prasaad(i)	Grace for All / by the Grace of

This saying expresses the attributes of the Divine and weaves a golden fabric of Sikh faith and philosophy. This practice of remembering the Lord, as taught by the Sikh gurus, does not take place externally, but goes out from within, in the form of constant awareness of the Name of the Divine. This name and truth cannot be comprehended rationally, but experienced by merging with it, through constant remembrance. The name—word—is to be remembered with full emotional sincerity, and in the deepest practice, it is coordinated with the breath.

In developing the aspirant's personality and eliminating barriers, the Sikh gurus also advised several cardinal virtues. These are: truth in action, contentment, compassion, fearlessness, humility, non-attachment, temperance, and the cultivation of wisdom. Guru Gobind Singh, the tenth guru, taught, established, and clarified the value of work as well as the contribution of 10% of one's income to the community welfare, and the idea of equality—of a congregation composed of equals. He established an executive council of five leaders to allow for decisions and instituted projects to ameliorate the lot of his congregation. When one loves his fellow man, he then sings praises of the Lord and as he sings and listens, his heart is transformed. When this occurs, then his mental outlook will also change. This constant remembrance of the Lord's name brings grace and the removal of all egoism and impurity. To rise, one must attune oneself to the higher Will, which is beyond the comprehension of mind and philosophy. Karmas done under the influence of ego only create further cause for death and rebirth, while the pure karmas of kirtan, remembrance, and service lead to reduction of ego and the ecstasy of union with the beloved.

Japa

Three methods of *japa* are taught: first, with the tongue, through *kirtan*, speaking, or chanting; second, in the mind, through mental repetition, and third, in the heart, by feeling the presence of the Lord within. When the practice becomes still deeper, then even the aspirant's very breath bears the name of the Divine. At the most advanced stage, the aspirant can think of nothing else. This is *ajapa japa*, or spontaneous remembrance. This process is achieved through the effort of the aspirant and the grace of guru and God.

The daily spiritual schedule of the Sikh was meant to help bring about this mindfulness. It involved rising and bathing, chanting *Japji* and meditating on the essence of the verses, going to the *gurdwara* (guru's home) for *darshana*, and the study of *Granth Sahib*, then listening to *kirtan* or *bani*, morning prayers. Then, the Sikh performed his worldly work and duties, ending the day with still more recitation and remembrance of the name of the Lord.

The five symbols used by the Sikhs *(kesh, kachha, kada, kangha,* and *kirpan)* are meant to help the Sikh maintain his mindfulness. *Kesh,* the long hair, signifies the maintenance of a saintly appearance and behavior in the midst of the world. *Kachha,* or the wearing of undergarments, symbolizes the practice of self-control and moderation. *Kada,* the steel bangle, reminds the Sikh to keep his physical actions pure and to refrain from theft, adultery or other distracting acts. *Kangha* (the comb), signifies purity and cleanliness on all levels, and *kirpan* (the sword) stands for fearlessness, determination, and will. These five symbols are meant on the physical level to help support the internal practice of *naam*, remembrance of the Lord's name.

India has long been the stronghold of sages such as Kabir, Tulsi Das, Sur Das, Tukaram, Sant Janeswar, Sri Ram Das, and many others, but Sri Guru Nanak Dev, the founder of Sikh dharma, was unique. The philosophy and faith of the most revered Nanak Dev has remained vibrant for hundreds of years. This is the evidence of the greatness of Sri Guru Nanak Dev. He has been a great source of inspiration to one and all. His teachings are ever fresh and evergreen for all times.

Sri Guru Nanak Dev (1469-1539), founder of the Sikh dharma, sought to establish harmony between diverse traditions and to make people aware that not tradition but truth should be followed with mind, action, and speech. He was a pioneer sage, who equally revered the fundamentals of all great religions, established a middle path, and rejected the non-essentials, embracing the path of love in a practical way. He is a singular example of his time. There are three words which explain the Sikh dharma in a nutshell: *guru*, *Granth*, and *Sikh*.

Guru is that great light which dispels the darkness of ignorance and is an exemplary spiritual guide. *Granth* consists of the sayings that record the Gurus' direct experience on the path of enlightenment, including moral, social, poetic, and spiritual teachings. A great poet and sage, who was filled with divine musical ecstasy, Guru Nanak Dev gives us a simple and profound teaching. These teachings, compiled by Sri Guru Arjan Dev, a successor in the guru lineage, are called the *Sri Granth Sahib,* in their compiled form.

The word *Granth* conveys that this is not like an ordinary book, but a compilation of beautiful teachings, just as one bead is set with others in a rosary. In exactly the same manner as this, the great sayings of Sri Nanak Dev and the other great sages were compiled into a text, which became a bible called *Granth Sahib*.

Sikh dharma, unlike other faiths, acknowledges the essential teachings of all the great religions but rejects the rigidity of ritual and useless religious observances, which consume time and energy and rob the chastity of human simplicity and endeavor.

The *Granth Sahib* was compiled by Sri Arjan Dev, the fifth guru, and it is called the *Adi Granth,* or the first book. It is written in a simple and poetic language, in a script called Gurmukhi, which means "that which emanates from the mouth of the perfect and Divine." Sikh dharma means that law that holds and sustains all in one, and the purpose of the Sikh dharma is to attain a state of supreme Consciousness by removing all differences and negativities between people, societies, and nations.

The word "dharma" has a different meaning than the word "religion." They are two separate institutions and concepts, which have distinct characteristics. Dharma is more profound, subtle, and practical, while religion is bound by temporal, dogmatic, and traditional rituals.

Truth, compassion, forgiveness, integrity, and selflessness are the hallmarks of "dharma." It is the source of humanity's finest virtues and values, the awareness of which removes all the barriers and reveals one's essential unity. The whole universe is a family and all the people are the members of one family.

In the annals of human history, there appears from time to time a great sage and leader who awakens the human heart's noblest qualities to such an extent that the nation changes its course of thinking, and thus, the entire society is directed toward God-consciousness, instead of ego-consciousness. Guru Nanak Dev was one such avatara, who restored self-respect to the downtrodden and humiliated masses of India and transformed the soul of a nation. Guru Nanak Dev thought that the mosque and the temple were equal in importance.

He expressed the brotherhood of humankind and had the goal of establishing harmonious relations between Hinduism and Islam. He embraced the universal principles of Hinduism and Sufism. No formalism, ritual, superstition, priesthood, dogma, mortification, or religious intolerance is found in the teachings of Guru Nanak

Dev. He refused to be lulled by the passivity of his times. He strove
to realize his ideal regardless of the cost. He valued devotion and
skillful action and not renunciation, and his goal was to uplift the
whole, not any one particular class or group.

The Sikh religion strives to create individuals who bring about
an ideal society that has as its basis spiritual awareness and ethical
integrity. The true Sikh is the householder who works hard to earn
a livelihood and gives to the world. Health and endurance of the
body, mind, and spirit are equally maintained; moderation, purity,
and selfless service are valued. Sikhism emphasizes the central unity
of religions, accepting the great words of diverse spiritual teachers
in a practical and synthesized way. Guru Nanak Dev said:

The throne of God exists in all places;
His treasure house fills up all spaces.
God, being Truth, lights up all faces.

In short, Sikhism expounds the ideal of a highly civilized
person who lives holistically, with inner awareness of the Lord and
with the purpose of serving the nation selflessly. Remembering the
name of the Lord of Life in every breath and studying the sacred
scriptures are the major spiritual practices. Guru Nanak Dev felt
that remembrance, harkening to the Name of the Lord, bestows
truth, divine wisdom, and contentment. Sikhism believes in one
God—formless, eternal, infinite, all-pervading, absolute, and beyond the comprehension of the human mind. Truth can be attained
by grace through devotion, righteousness, and selfless service. This
is similar to the teachings of Vedanta, the last and finest part of the
Vedas, though expressed in a simple and lucid manner. The *Vedas*
and the *Upanishads* are not understood by the common people,
while the sayings of the *Granth Sahib* can be understood, practiced,
and followed by anyone and everyone.

Guru Nanak Dev taught that for man to be saved, he must live
according to the Truth. He should not keep feelings of animosity
for anyone. Forgiveness is love at its highest power. He taught that
forgiveness is God Himself. A great humanist, he advocated

equality, devotion, and service as principal tenets of his path. He valued *ahimsa*, non-harming, as a guideline for action and instructed his followers to practice it.

Guru Nanak Dev was the son of Hindu parents who lived near Lahore (now in Pakistan). In his youth, he sought out the company of wandering hermits before establishing himself in the life of a householder. He was preoccupied with spiritual matters, studying the devotional literature, especially the writings of Kabir and several other sages, and of the Sufis. For thirty years he dedicated himself fulltime to spirituality, traveling with his disciples, Bala and Mardana. Eventually, he settled in Kartarpur, where he resumed the householder's life in an exemplary way. The last fifteen years of his life were spent teaching his disciples. The universality and vitality of his teachings revived the true essence of spirituality in India.

Guru Nanak Dev instituted the lineage of gurus by designating his disciple, Sri Angad Dev (1504-1552) as his successor, thereby setting aside his own son, who believed in the path of renunciation and ascetic practices. His successor, Sri Angad Dev, chose his elderly disciple Sri Amar Das (1479-1574), a great reformer, to succeed him as the third guru. Guru Amar Das helped to improve the position of women by abolishing *purdah* (veiling) and *sati pratha* (self-immolation of widows). He made communal dining of all his followers mandatory, without any discrimination on the basis of caste, creed, or color. He was succeeded by his son-in-law Guru Ram Das (1534-1581), founder of the holy city of Amritsar.

Guru Ram Das's youngest son, Sri Arjan Dev (1563-1606), the fifth guru, made Amritsar a place of pilgrimage by installing there the *Adi Granth*, which he compiled and to which he contributed. He built many temples throughout the Punjab.

Guru Arjan Dev's son, Guru Har Govind (1595-1644), channeled the Sikh desire to regain the prestige and dignity of the people by uniting them through training in arms. His disciplined valor became characteristic of the Sikh disciples, who rallied devotedly around their guru and became the defenders of dharma. His successor, Sri Har Rai (1630-1661), continued to acquire arms and train warriors to repel tyranny and injustice. Sri Har Rai's son, Sri Harkrishan (1656-1664), the eighth Sikh guru, served only three years, and despite his youth wisely selected a worthy and deserving successor, Sri Tegh Bahadur (1621-1675), thus also bypassing several relatives to do so.

Guru Tegh Bahadur, the ninth guru, was a wise and strong leader who had lived in isolation for a long time before assuming leadership. He then traveled widely to convey the Sikh teachings throughout the country. He founded Anandpur in the Shivalik Hills, which provided a more secure position than did the plains surrounding Amritsar. He was also a poet, as had been the first five gurus. He fathered Gobind Rai, who was to become Guru Gobind Singh, the last guru, glorious and unparalleled in human history, a combination of sage, poet, warrior, and a leader.

Sikh Dharma

Dharma is the very source of philosophical conclusions. Sikh dharma is based on the sayings of *Granth Sahib*, which is one of the most highly philosophical, devotional, and practical bibles in the library of man today. Scholars only discuss and repeat the same thing again and again, reducing this great universal dharma to mere religious observances. All the Research Foundations on Sri Nanak Dev's work should take up and investigate such projects as the "socialism" of Sikhism, the psychology of Sikhism, the philosophy of Sikhism, and spirituality in Sikhism.

It was a great loss, not just to the Sikh community, but to all learned and literary persons, that a vast amount of literature, especially many rare manuscripts, was destroyed during the Blue Star operation. Temples and gurdwaras can be rebuilt with bricks, but this irreparable loss can never be recovered. The historians should sit down once again and rethink the writings on the aspects of Sikhism which are not yet tapped by writers, poets, and singers.

The delay in my completion of rendering the *Granth Sahib* in rhyming verse is due to many hurdles, one of which is my limited knowledge of the ragas mentioned in *Granth Sahib*. I am making sincere efforts to correctly put forward this version of the *Granth*

Sahib in rhyming verse so that the readers do not have any difficulty with it. I have all the English, Gurmukhi, Hindi, and Urdu versions of *Granth Sahib*. My knowledge of Gurmukhi, however, is poor, and off and on, I seek advice from scholars of Gurmukhi. After rhyming *Sri Japji*, I recently completed rhyming *Sri Sukhamani Sahib*, one of the great books of the Sikh tradition.

Recently, political socialism in Sikh dharma is being propagated, ignoring the very foundation of Sikh faith and philosophy. The result is that the Sikh community and Sikh dharma are not rightly understood. In India today, every Sikh is painted as a terrorist. I know many devoted Sikhs who lead householder lives and yet are like highly evolved sages. There is presently a lack of dynamic leadership however, and for lack of a leader, the problem is determining who will follow whom, for everyone wants to become a leader. I am writing this the way I feel, see, and observe, as there have been conferences and gatherings in the congregation in the past. Why do we not continue to hold such gatherings and conferences? Why do the scholars of Sikhism not communicate and interact by being creative and giving something to the weary and torn masses of India and the world?

All the great religions are given by the one and the same Source, and you can term that as Truth, God, or Providence, but the Sikh dharma has so much to offer and yet the scriptures have not been widely circulated, especially in the English, French, German, Italian, or Spanish languages. Thus, people outside India do not understand much about the Sikhs.

There is another point that I want to mention: in many ways the style and way of life that a Sikh commonly leads are positively superior to anyone of any religion. Recently, however, Sikhs have been isolating themselves, and isolation leads to the rigidity of contraction, while the Sikh dharma teaches expansion. Sometimes a superiority complex misleads a person, community, or nation, and thus, the values of a great dharma are misinterpreted, distorted, or misrepresented by its followers. What happened to Hinduism and Hindu society, when the great scriptures were not properly interpreted or communicated so that they could be understood and followed by the common masses? The multiplicity of shrines has destroyed the great ancient pillars of the teachings.

Guru Nanak Dev was able to create a golden bridge between the two traditions, cultures, and religions of Hinduism and Islam. India has been a melting pot throughout the ages. Unfortunately, Indians do not know how to create a coherence among the different factions of society, religion, and faith. This is one of the greatest truths, which even Tagore, Gandhiji and others could not accomplish. This does not mean, however, that if something has not been accomplished that we should not continue to make efforts. Numerous flowers of different species can bloom in one garden. A million stars can twinkle in the sky without interfering with each other's light. If the sun and moon can shine and pale their lights, then why cannot harmony be established in the Punjab in India? This is a question that constantly erodes the edges of my heart.

This book, *Philosophy and Faith of Sikhism,* will help the English-knowing readers to have a glimpse of the Sikh community and philosophy. Those who do not know anything about the Sikhs will also come to understand some things about their tradition.

Dr. K. S. Duggal, a great and creative writer, and a real Sikh, has beautifully explained in this book the great gems of Truth that are laid down in the Sikh dharma. I am sure this book will be of great benefit to the reader.

Swami Rama

Introduction

Modern India has a secular constitution where the law of the land equally respects all religions.

Mahatma Gandhi, father of the nation, was a Hindu and yet he studied and venerated other religions whose hymns were regularly recited at his prayer-meetings. These included Buddhism, Jainism, Christianity, Islam, Zoroastrianism, and Sikhism. Jawaharlal Nehru professed himself a non-believer and yet he visited places of worship with the apparent devotion of his countrymen. He was invested with the sacred thread as a child and Vedic ceremonials were duly observed at his cremation and to his memory. Mrs. Indira Gandhi's spiritual thirst carried her to any locale where she could find peace of mind, whether at a Hindu, Muslim, or Sikh holy place.

Within this context of many religions, Sikhism is the most modern, the most recent, and the most scientific faith amongst the great religions of the world. Its founder, Guru Nanak, had the advantage of having drunk deep at the founts of all the sacred religious lore. A life-long pilgrim, he visited the ancient Hindu temple at Puri in the east, Holy Mecca in the west, the ascetics at Manasarovar deep into the Himalayas in the north, and in the south the Buddhist shrines in Sri Lanka. Venerated equally by the Hindus and the Muslims in the Punjab, he is still remembered as *Baba Nanak Shah faqir / Hindu da guru, Musalman da pir* (a great Sufi, revered *guru* of Hindus, *pir* of Muslims).

Guru Nanak lived through the harrowing experience of a Mughal invasion of the Punjab by Babar. This cruel invader murdered, raped, and recklessly destroyed property. The poet in Guru Nanak fearlessly condemned the atrocities committed by the

Mughal forces. For a moment, it seems, he revolted even against divine justice. Said he:

> Ati mar pai kurlanen!
> Tainki dard no aiya?
> (Such suffering and such wailing!
> Did it not hurt you?)

(Asa)

And yet never, never in his voluminous writing did Guru Nanak utter a word against Islam. He decried the Turks and the Pathans who attacked his country but never the Muslims who were as much his countrymen as were the Hindus. On the other hand, while undertaking a pilgrimage to Holy Mecca, he is said to have donned the blue robes of the Muslim pilgrims:

> Neel bastar lai kapde pehre
> Turk Pathani amal kiya
> (He wore the blue robes
> The way a Turk or a Pathan does.)

(Asa di Var)

And yet for Guru Nanak, who was born a Hindu, communal harmony was a creed which he supported vigorously throughout his life.

Guru Gobind Singh, the creator of the Khalsa, had the unique distinction of combining in himself the guru and the disciple. He baptized the Sikhs and then sat at their feet to be baptized by them. An ardent democrat in his social behavior, he many times declared that he owed all his glory to his people *(Inhi ki kripa se saje ham hain)*. At the close of his ministry, he invested his authority as a guru, both temporal and secular, in the *panth,* the five elected representatives—*the Panj Piaras.*

The current tension among Hindus and Sikhs in the Punjab, though unfortunate in the extreme, is no new phenomenon. It raises its head periodically when mischievous elements in the population gain undue influence. Clearly there is a need for Sikhs to maintain a unique identity. A few decades ago, the Sikhs had to shout from the house-tops—*Hum Hindu nahin hain* (We are not Hindus). Such declarations were used to ward off a real or imaginary attack on their identity. At that time as great a poet and patriot as Puran Singh came forward and said:

"The great Hindu culture and its innate influence on Sikh culture cannot be denied.

"The Sikh is in no sense an alien, he is born in India, he has the glorious heritage of Indian culture, he cannot be without Prahlad and Mira. Guru Gobind Singh sent his Sikhs to Banaras to study Sanskrit. He is said to have translated *Krishna Lila* himself.

"Our mother-country is India, our language is derived from Sanskrit, but we are modern in outlook, though also ancient as Prahlad and Krishna.

"In view of the political solidarity of India it is mischievous for anyone to suggest that we are not Hindus, and not equally Muslims. It is mischievous to multiply the points of difference with the Hindus, which are not fundamental."

What seems to bother the Sikhs currently is again the question of their identity. There are many front-rank intellectuals in the community who fear that with the onslaught of modernism, the Sikhs may be swept off their feet and lose their identity. Nothing could be farther from the truth. If the gatherings of the devotees at the Sikh Gurdwaras are any indication, the faith in the Sikh way of life is growing every day. Gurdwara Bangla Sahib in Delhi, which used to be a quiet shrine a few decades ago, is now crowded with devotees at all hours. The same is true of other Sikh holy places throughout the country. And we have among the Sikhs many people who would be willing to make any sacrifice for the preservation of the Sikh tradition.

The Sikhs have for the first time in history a State in which they are in the majority and where Punjabi is the main language.

This is something which even the great Maharaja Ranjit Singh could not claim for the community. It is time to make the best of this opportunity rather than fritter away the fund of the community's energies in vain pursuits.

I hurriedly wrote this book to respond to the mounting tension in the Punjab which started with the clash between the Akali and Nirankari factions at Amritsar and then spread to embroil the entire State. Inevitably this tension has taken the all too familiar form of community versus community.

The Sikhs are a "spirit-born people" who have a noble heritage which would give pride to any community. They are hard-working and enterprising. They are friendly and forward-looking, imbued with a rare spirit of self-sacrifice. It is their endeavor mainly that has helped the country turn the corner in food production. Guarding a sensitive border, they are the virtual sword-arm of India. Their contribution in the freedom struggle is unique. Their sacrifices are legendary in various conflicts with intruders into independent India, whether they came from the north-east or the north-west. They are always in the forefront of every national endeavor. It hardly becomes a people with their great past and no less glorious present to tarnish their image with narrow and parochial considerations.

Part of this text was previously published in *The Tribune,* a leading newspaper of the Punjab. It is hoped that this book will serve all readers in India and abroad so that they understand the great Sikh tradition with all its profundities.

The
Sikh Tradition

1.

A Messiah of Amity and Integration

Baba Nanak, the great man of God
Is the guru of the Hindu
and the pir of the Musalman.

This is how the Hindus and the Muslims in the Punjab came to remember Guru Nanak. It is said, when he died, the Hindus wanted to cremate him and the Muslims insisted on burying him. It is no wonder, since during his lifetime he visited Hardwar, Varanasi, and Puri as a devout Hindu would do. He also went on pilgrimage to Mecca and Medina donning the blue garments of a Turk or a Pathan. He made friends with *siddhas*—Hindu ascetics— and had prolonged dissertations with them. He also cultivated Muslim divines and mystics and discoursed with them on the ways of man and God. For his constant companions he had Mardana, a Muslim *rabab*-player, and Bala, a Hindu, who is said to be the author of his earliest biography, called *Janam Sakhi Bhai Bala*. Guru Nanak knew Persian and wrote poetry in it. He was equally proficient in Sanskrit and could claim scholarship in the *Vedas* and the *Shastras*. His was indeed an integrated personality without equal, rare in the annals of human history.

Even as a child, Guru Nanak started rejecting one after another the superstitious practices, meaningless ceremonials, and anti- quated rituals current in the society of his day. His directness annoyed many, including his own father. He exasperated the Hindu priest and was the despair of the Muslim *maulvi*. At an early age, his own sister Bibi Nanaki and the Muslim chief of the village, Rai Bular, noticed remarkable signs of divinity in Guru

3

Nanak. It is still being debated among theologians as to who was the first to give allegiance to the Master—his sister Bibi Nanaki or Rai Bular, the village headman.

Guru Nanak condemned hypocrisy and ritualism whether he found it in Hinduism or Islam. He believed in clean, honest living with faith in one God. He looked around and said, "There is no Hindu; there is no Musalman." He wanted Hindus to be good Hindus and Muslims to be good Muslims. He insisted that Islam or Hinduism did not consist of mere exterior forms and hollow rituals.

According to a custom prevalent among caste Hindus, Guru Nanak was to be invested with a sacred thread. It is a sacrament like baptism among the Christians, signifying the spiritual rebirth of a Hindu child. When the family priest approached the young Nanak, he refused to wear the "cotton thread." He had no faith in this ritual. He would have nothing to do with a thread which must wear out sooner or later. Said Guru Nanak:

> Let mercy be the cotton, contentment the thread,
> Continence the knot and truth the twist,
> O Priest! if you have such a sacred thread,
> Do give it to me.
> It'll not wear out, nor get soiled,
>   nor be burnt, nor lost.
> Says Nanak, blessed are those who
>   wear a thread like this.

(Asa)

Once the Nawab of Sultanpur and his *qazi* invited Guru Nanak to say prayers with them. Guru Nanak had no objection. He was willing to keep company with those who had faith in God. However, when they commenced the prayers, Guru Nanak stood aside and watched them with a smile on his lips. As soon as the prayers were over, the *qazi* asked Guru Nanak, "Why didn't you join us in prayers after agreeing to do so?"

Guru Nanak told him politely, "I did not join you because all the while you were saying the prayers, your mind was on your filly left loose back at your place. You feared that she might fall into the well in your courtyard." The *qazi* heard it and was silenced. "In that case, you could have given me your company," said the Nawab. "But you were buying horses in Kabul," observed Guru Nanak. The Nawab realized the truth of it. At this Guru Nanak said:

> Let God's grace be the mosque,
> and devotion the prayer-mat,
> Let *Quran* be the good conduct,
> Let modesty be compassion, good manners fasting,
> You should be a Musalman the like of this.
> Let good deeds be your Kaaba and
> truth be your mentor.
> Your *Kalma* be your creed and prayer.
> God would then vindicate your honor.

> *(Majh)*

It is no wonder that well-meaning Hindus and Muslims both held Guru Nanak in great esteem. The Muslim treated him as *Waliallah*—a beloved of God— and until recently a large number of Hindus in the Punjab followed the teachings of Guru Nanak and had at least one child in the family baptized as a Sikh.

During his lifetime, Guru Nanak undertook several journeys to the north, south, east, and west with a view to spreading his message of the brotherhood of man and the unity of God. In the east, he went as far as Nagaland. In the south, he visited even Sri Lanka and Lakshadweep. In the north, he crossed Kashmir and penetrated deep into the Himalayas as far as Mansarovar, meeting ascetics who had withdrawn themselves from the world. And in the west, there is historical evidence that he went as far as Baghdad. All these arduous journeys helped in fostering understanding and amity. Wherever he went, he is remembered and revered even today.

While journeying towards the east, Guru Nanak is said to have visited Gorakhmata, a shrine devoted to Gorakh Nath, not very far from Pilibhit. The ascetics here argued fiercely with Guru Nanak, but they were, at last, completely won over. Their center came to be known as Nanakmata. It is a place of pilgrimage even today. This is what Guru Nanak told them:

> Asceticism doesn't lie in the ascetic robes,
> Nor in the walking staff, nor in the ashes.
> Asceticism doesn't lie in the earring,
> Nor in the shaven head, nor in blowing a conch.
> Asceticism lies in remaining pure amidst impurities.
>
> *(Suhi)*

On his way back from Assam, Guru Nanak returned *via* Orissa visiting the famous temple of Jagannath at Puri. It is one of the most important places of Hindu pilgrimage. Guru Nanak found that the priests of the temple attached more importance to rituals than to true faith in God. Throughout the day these priests made elaborate arrangements with perfumed trays of flowers and burning candles in order to propitiate the deity. They called it *arati*. But none of the devotees joining the ritual had his heart in it. Guru Nanak withdrew from the empty ritual and, sitting outside the temple, starting singing, Mardana accompanying him on the *rabab*:

> The sky is the tray,
> The sun and the moon are the lights
> And the stars the jewels.
> Sandalwood's fragrance is the incense,
> The wind is the fly-whisk
> And all the forests your flowers.
> What a wonderful *arati* it is!
>
> *(Dhanasri)*

In the meantime, the priests and pilgrims had collected around Guru Nanak and they were thrilled to hear him sing the praises of God.

When Guru Nanak arrived at Mecca, he felt tired. It had been a long and strenuous journey to the holy city. He fell asleep and it so happened that he slept with his feet towards Kaaba, the holy shrine, instead of his head, which was the accepted practice. At midnight, Jiwan, the watchman, on his rounds noticed this and was scandalized to find a pilgrim with his feet pointing towards the House of God. "How dare you lie with your feet pointing towards God?" he shouted. He was about to lay his corrective hands on Nanak when the Guru woke up. "My good man, I am weary after a long journey. Kindly turn my feet in the direction where God is not." Jiwan was stunned. "Where God is not!" His head started whirling. "Where God is not!" He saw His abode in all four directions. He had lifted Nanak's feet and rather than turning them around, his head fell on them. He started kissing them. He washed Guru Nanak's feet with his tears.

The other pilgrims and the holy men of the shrine were delighted to have Guru Nanak amidst them. They asked him many questions. "I am neither a Hindu nor a Musalman," said Guru Nanak. "Who is superior of the two?" the pilgrims collected around him wished to know. Guru Nanak replied, "Without good deeds, neither is good." The Guru laid stress on the love of God, humility, prayer, and truthful living. He then recited a hymn in Persian:

> I beseech You, O Lord! pray grant me a hearing.
> You are the truthful, the great, the merciful,
>   and the faultless Creator.
> I know for certain, this world must perish,
> And death must come, I know this and nothing else.
> Neither wife, nor son, nor father, nor brother
>   shall be able to help.
> I must go in the end, none could undo
>   what is written in my lot.
> I have spent days and nights in vanity
>   contemplating evil.
> Never have I thought of good; this is what I am,

I am ill-starred, miserly, careless,
    short-sighted and rude.
But I am yours,
    the dust of the feet of your minions.

(Tilang)

Guru Nanak's most vehement disapproval was directed toward the caste system that had petrified Hindu society since time immemorial. A person born in a low caste was condemned to all sorts of discrimination in life. And after years of exposure, the virus of the caste system had inevitably penetrated into Muslim society as well. There were *Syeds* and *Maulvis, Sheikhs* and *Mussallis* among them. Guru Nanak would have none of it.

Early in his life Guru Nanak happened to visit Saidpur. He chose to stay with Bhai Lalo, a carpenter. It so happened that the day Guru Nanak arrived, Malik Bhago, the chief of the town, who had amassed untold wealth, was holding a sacrificial feast to which all the holy men were invited. Guru Nanak decided to remain away and partook of the simple fare of his host. When Malik Bhago came to know of it, he was furious. Guru Nanak didn't care a bit. As for worldly wealth, he maintained:

It cannot be collected without unfair means
And when you die, it doesn't go with you.

Unlike Mahavira and Buddha, Nanak was not born to affluent parents. He was the son of a village *patwari,* at the lowest rung of the revenue hierarchy. While playing in the company of children he always made friends with the poor and the so-called low castes. After his Revelation at Sultanpur, he had a simple message for all who came to see him: One must work and share one's earnings with others, and an active life is superior to a contemplative life.

His sympathies were always with the poor and the have-nots. He suffered with suffering humanity. During Babar's invasion of India, Guru Nanak witnessed frightful killings. The poet in him seems to have revolted against divine justice. Guru Nanak has left a remarkable piece of poetry describing the barbarous attack and the sufferings of the people of the Punjab:

> He occupied Khurasan and subdued Hindustan,
> God! Don't You blame yourself for having
>   sent the Mughal like a doom?
> Seeing such killing and wailing,
>   didn't it hurt You, O Lord?
> You are the lone Creator of all.
> If an aggressor were to kill an aggressor
> I wouldn't complain.
> But when a fierce lion falls on
>   a poor herd of cattle
> The master must take the blame. . . .
>
>   *(Asa)*

It required a great deal of courage to say all this about a foreign invader who was determined to settle down and found an empire. *Babarvani* has a number of other composition, which also condemn both the invader and the Godless, corrupt Hindu society of the day that had invited trouble on itself:

> They who had beautiful locks and the
>   vermilion dye in the parting of their hair
> Have their tresses shorn with scissors and
>   dust thrown on their heads.
> They wouldn't remember Ram
> They can't take the name of Allah now.
>
>   *(Asa)*

During the close of his ministry, Guru Nanak settled down at Kartarpur on the banks of the river Ravi. It was a new township established by the Guru himself on a tract of land placed at his disposal by one of his followers. Here all the residents, including Guru Nanak, shared the work, tilled the land, and ate from a common kitchen. It is said that Kartarpur was the first ever experiment in community living. Khushwant Singh observes in his *History of the Sikhs:*

"The *bhaktas* had paid only lip service to the ideal of casteless society, Nanak took practical steps to break the vicious hold of caste by starting a free community kitchen—*Guru Ka Langar*—in all centers and persuading his followers, irrespective of their castes, to eat together."

Guru Nanak identified himself with the lowest of the low. He refers to himself as "Nanak, the servant," "Nanak, the low-caste," "Nanak, the humble." Integration is best ensured when the man at the top starts from the bottom. Says Guru Nanak:

Among the low, let my caste be the lowest.
Of the lowly, let me the lowliest be.
O Nanak, let such be the men I know,
With such men let me keep company.
Why must I try to emulate the great?

(Majh)

2.

In the Footsteps of the Master

He ascended the throne of Guru Nanak,
The Guru's spirit entering the disciple.

This is how Bhai Gurdas, one of the earliest Sikh chroniclers, describes Guru Angad's installation as the second Sikh Guru. Tradition holds that on being named a successor, the divine light of Guru Nanak enters. And so it has occurred with each successor, one after the other. Accordingly, each successor has adopted the name of Nanak and written under that name.

Guru Angad, the first successor, found that he had inherited a magnificent tradition of communal love and understanding. Unlike other *bhaktas, sufis,* and saints, Guru Nanak did not take a simplistic view of communal harmony. He did not intend a superficial synthesis of Hinduism and Islam. It was not a case of reevaluation, rejecting some and accepting some other features in either faith and then blending them. More than horizontal intermingling, which did have its virtues, Guru Nanak laid stress on the vertical elevation of society and the spiritual coalescing of the two communities. He wanted Hindus to be good Hindus and Muslims to be good Muslims. Wherever he went, he set up *manjis*, where his followers could congregate regularly, both Hindus and Muslims, and remember God.

Guru Nanak had also rejected Sanskrit and Persian for communication. He opted for the language of the people, accepting all local dialects. Adopting the local dialect brought him closer to the people. Propagation of the mother-tongue obliterated differences in the various communities and provided them with a common bond. A common language can be a mighty unifying force. The Hindus were drifting away to Sanskrit and the Muslims were taking to Persian more and more. *Bhaktas* like Guru Nanak helped stem this tendency. The gulf was bridged to a great extent. The protagonists of the Bhakti Movement evolved a way of com- munication called *sadhukari*, spoken and popularized by the poet- saints in medieval times. It is exactly like a language called *sandhya bhasa*, which is a language spoken among highly evolved yogis and sages.

Not only this, Guru Nanak adopted poetic forms that were popular with the people at large. Their meters and measures followed the folksongs and folk ballads that the common people were familiar with. Guru Nanak tried *Siharfi, Baramah, Kafi* and several other molds popular with Muslims as also *Chhanda, Ashtapadi, Doha* and *Sloka* in the best tradition of Hindu classical poetry. He drew his similes from the everyday life of the common man. He employed familiar symbols like the spinning-wheel, the bride and the parents' house, always with a fresh approach.

Since it is easy to remember poetry, and easier to convey it by word of mouth, all the writings that Guru Nanak has bequeathed to his followers are in verse. Not only this, almost all his poetry can be sung to music. The text conforms to specific *ragas* prevalent in the Hindustani style of music of the day. Where Guru Nanak followed better-known musical forms of folk ballads, he made it a point to mention the fact in the beginning of the composition, that it was designed to be sung in a certain tune in the style of a specific ballad. For instance, in the opening of *Asa di Var*, a long work sung by the Sikh community every morning as a divine service, it is stated:

"The *Var* with *slokas* is written by the First Guru
and should be sung to the air of *Tunda Asraja*."

Guru Nanak played many roles in his life. He was a recluse, an ascetic and a family man who married and had children. He was devoted to his sister. He was a dutiful husband. He was a loving father. And yet he was not excessively attached to anyone. When the time came to nominate his successor, Guru Nanak felt that neither of his sons were qualified for the honor. This was the greatest test of his life. His sons aspired to succeed him. One of them had never married and had lived the life of an ascetic. Guru Nanak did not approve of it. He attached greater importance to normal family life. Therefore, he ordained one of his followers as the next Guru. Lehna by name, he was blessed by Nanak with his *ang* (hand) and he became Guru Angad.

It is told that Malu Shah, an orderly in the Mughal army, came to Guru Angad for spiritual guidance. The Guru was aware that the Mughals were experiencing difficulties during those days. He advised Malu Shah to remain loyal to his master and serve his King devotedly, all the more so during the King's adversity.

Humayun had succeeded Babar on the Mughal throne but he was soon overpowered by Sher Shah. As Humayun was being routed, he came over to Khadur to seek Guru Angad's blessings. It so happened that, when he arrived, the Guru was sitting in a congregation listening to hymns being sung by the devotees. Therefore the Mughal King had to wait for a while. Humayun felt slighted and, losing his temper, put his hand on the hilt of his sword, threatening to attack the Guru. Guru Angad remained unperturbed and calm as ever. He chided Humayun: "When you should have used the sword, you did not, rather you ran away from the battlefield like a coward. Here with a dervish, you show off, threatening to attack unarmed devotees engaged in prayer." Humayun heard this and was full of remorse. He wished to be pardoned. Guru Angad reminded him about Guru Nanak's prophecy:

"They come in '78 and go in '97. Another man of the sword will also arise."*

*The prophecy relates to the Mughals occupying India in Samvat 1578 (1521 A.D.) and departing in Samvat 1597 (1540 A.D.). The monarch who was driven out was Humayun, and the "man of the sword" refered to is Sher Shah, who had thrown him out.

The Guru told him that he must leave the country in his own interest and that, as foreseen by the Great Guru, he would return to his throne shortly thereafter. History is witness that Humayun attacked India in due course and regained his throne.

Guru Angad was fond of children and took great interest in them. He gathered children together, organized games for them and distributed prizes. He also devoted considerable attention to their proper education. He insisted that children should be taught in their mother-tongue and to that end he is said to have simplified and codified the Gurmukhi script, and popularized its use among the Sikhs. This, perhaps, is the most important contribution of Guru Angad. While the origin of the Gurmukhi script continues to be disputed, there is no doubt that Guru Angad was a leader in making extensive use of this script. He commissioned a number of copies of Guru Nanak's *bani* to be made in Gurmukhi script, which consists of thirty-five letters.

When the time came for Guru Angad to name his successor, he installed Guru Amar Das, one of his devotees, as the next Guru. Guru Angad's two sons didn't like the decision. They had their own ambitions. Guru Angad told them that the honor must go to the one who deserved it most.

Said Satta, a bard of the Guru's household:

> "The brotherhood was delighted to see Guru Nanak's umbrella over Amar Das's head."

Guru Angad was seventy-three when Guru Amar Das was ordained. A mere devotee who prided himself on being the humblest servant of the Guru, he lived where the Guru desired him to live, and did what the Guru asked him to do. He was then raised to the supreme status of a Master who provided leadership to innumerable followers near and far.

Guru Nanak had laid stress on *sangat*. The Sikhs must congregate both in the morning and evening and sing praises of the Almighty. Guru Amar Das streamlined the practice by setting up twenty-two *manjis* (dioceses) formally presided over by devout

Sikhs. With a view to spreading Guru Nanak's message far and wide, he trained a band of one hundred forty-six apostles, of whom fifty-two were women, to go to the various parts of the country and attend to the spiritual needs of the Guru's followers.

However, Guru Amar Das's most distinguished contribution was the concept of *pangat.* The idea was that Sikhs must sit and eat together. He set up a free kitchen where everyone, irrespective of caste and creed, was welcome. In fact, the Guru made it obligatory on all those seeking his audience, first to eat in the *langar* and then to see him. This helped in ridding Hindu society of the evils of the caste system and brought the Hindus and the Muslims closer, thereby fostering communal harmony. The Guru also tried to eradicate social evils like *sati,* which required a Hindu widow to either burn herself on her husband's funeral pyre or to remain unmarried for the rest of her life.

As the message of Guru Nanak spread, more and more people visited Goindwal, the city established by Guru Amar Das. It became a flourishing town and a number of Muslim dignitaries also came and settled there.

During one of his visits to Lahore, the Emperor Akbar was crossing the river Beas. He decided to make a slight detour and visit Goindwal to pay homage to Guru Amar Das about whom he had heard a great deal. To see the Guru, even the Emperor had to partake of food in the *langar* like any other visitor. It is said that even the Emperor sat with the lowliest of the low, ate with them, and then had his audience with the Guru. Akbar was highly impressed and wished to grant a *jagir* to the Guru for the maintenance of the free kitchen. The Guru would not agree to it. "We start afresh every morning. Nothing is saved for the next day," said the Guru. "The rations are brought by the devotees daily and are distributed among them every day." The Emperor insisted upon making the grant in appreciation of the great humanitarian work being done by the Guru. Since the Guru would not accept any favor from the King, Akbar thought of a way out. "I can, at least, present a few villages as a wedding gift to your daughter, Bhani, who is as much my daughter." The Guru could not decline it and the King had his way. It was at this spot that Amritsar, the renowned Sikh center, came to be established in due course.

It is said that the orthodox Hindus complained to the King that Guru Amar Das was violating their time-honored practices by rejecting Sanskrit and criticizing their rituals and religious practices. The Guru listened to the King's suggestions in the interest of communal harmony and agreed to visit Hindu holy places. He found God everywhere. The King, on his part, went out of his way to exempt the Guru and his followers from the pilgrim tax. It is said, wherever the Guru went, he attracted large crowds. The Guru's slogan, *Sat Nam Sri Waheguru,* resounded everywhere.

"You are Nanak, you are Lehna, you are Amar Das," Satta the bard sang when Guru Ram Das succeeded as the fourth Sikh Guru. Guru Ram Das's ministry was short-lived, a period of only seven year. After he had been ordained as the Guru, Guru Ram Das (who was the son-in-law of Guru Amar Das) started building a new township on the *jagir* granted to his wife Bibi Bhani by Akbar. This new township is what came to be known as Amritsar. The name Amritsar is derived from the holy tank called Amritsar—the pool of nectar, around which the town grew.

Guru Ram Das wanted to provide the community with a nucleus, but he could neither complete the holy tank nor start constructing the Golden Temple on its present site because rather early in life, he handed over the stewardship of the community to his youngest son Guru Arjan Dev, a sensitive poet and an eminent scholar.

About Guru Arjan, his own grandfather, Guru Amar Das had said:

> "This grandson of mine will cruise people across the ocean of life."

Though Guru Amar Das had indicated beyond any doubt that Guru Arjan Dev would be ordained the Guru in due course, his eldest brother Prithi Chand, was never reconciled to this decision, and he created considerable trouble. He started scheming and conspiring against the Guru. Guru Arjan didn't take much notice of him for he was busy completing a number of undertakings left unfinished by Guru Ram Das.

Guru Arjan had the foundation-stone of *Harimandir*, later know as the Golden Temple, laid by Mian Mir, a Muslim divine of Lahore. The Sikhs desired that it should be the tallest building in town. The Guru, however, thought otherwise. He reminded his followers that there was no virtue like humility. The temple was, therefore, built on as low an elevation as possible. He also decided to have the new temple open on all four sides. Anyone could enter it from any side. No one might be discriminated against.

As he was busy attending to the construction of the Holy Tank and the Holy Temple, reports came to Guru Arjan that Prithi Chand, his eldest brother had started composing his own hymns and was passing them to the Sikhs visiting Amritsar as the compositions of Guru Nanak and other Sikh Gurus. If this was allowed, Guru Arjan feared it would be the undoing of the faith. He therefore decided to compile an authentic text of hymns that he and the four preceding Gurus had composed. The compilation when completed came to be known as the *Holy Granth*. Consistent with the tradition of the Sikh faith, Guru Arjan had a number of spiritual verses composed by other Indian saints, both Hindu and Muslim, collected and included in the compilation. It was a rare act of communal amity for which it is hard to find a parallel.

However, Prithi Chand was not to be deterred. He complained to the Mughal Court that the *Holy Granth* had derogatory references to Muslim and Hindu prophets and saints. Akbar had the *Granth* examined and found there was no truth in the charges. He was delighted to be acquainted with the highly inspiring volume. He bestowed robes of honor on the Sikhs who had carried the *Holy Granth* to him and sent numerous gifts to the Guru. He also promised to pay his respects personally to the Guru the next time he visited Lahore.

The Emperor kept his promise and went on pilgrimage to Amritsar. He was greatly impressed with the activities of the Guru.

He made rich offerings and sought the Guru's blessing for the peace and welfare of his Kingdom. At the Guru's intervention he exempted the region from the land tax, as it had suffered a severe drought that year. Unfortunately, a monarch of vision like Akbar did not live long. He was followed on the throne by his son Jehangir, though Akbar had nominated his grandson, Khusro, to succeed him.

Jehangir was a pleasure-loving man given to drinking. He left the administration of the Kingdom to his Queen and his courtiers. While on his way to Kashmir, the Emperor Jehangir summoned Guru Arjan to meet him at Lahore. He asked the Guru to revise the *Holy Granth* deleting all references to Islam and Hinduism. How could the Guru agree to it? He was, therefore, fined two lakhs of rupees. The Guru told the king that his money was the sacred trust of the Sikh community and the hymns in the *Holy Granth* were a revelation in praise of God; no one dare alter them. The King was on his way to Kashmir. He was in a hurry and in no mood to involve himself in an argument.

In the meanwhile the *qazi* gave his injunction ordering the Guru to be tortured to death, in case he did not agree to expunge the so-called derogatory references to Islam and Hinduism contained in the *Holy Granth*. It is said that the Guru was forced to sit on a sheet of red hot iron. They poured hot sand on his body. He was then lowered into boiling water. As the Guru was being persecuted in this manner, he was visited by Mian Mir, the Muslim divine of Lahore who had laid the foundation-stone of the Holy Temple at Amritsar. Mir begged the Guru to allow him to use his mystic powers to undo those who were responsible for the suffering inflicted upon the Guru. Guru Arjan heard Mian Mir but counseled patience. He told him that one must accept the will of God; not a leaf moves if God doesn't ordain it.

The Guru was tortured for five days. When Jehangir's soldiers found him bearing all the agony with perfect equanimity, they became helpless. They were at a loss to know what to do. At this moment, the Guru asked to take a bath in the river Ravi which ran by the side of the Mughal fort in which he was imprisoned. As thousands of his followers watched with tears in their eyes, the Guru walked to the river. His bare body glistened with blisters. There were blisters on his feet and he couldn't even walk properly. "Sweet is Your will, O God; the gift of Your name alone I seek," said the Guru again and again. As he reached the river, he bade farewell to his devotees and walked into the water as serene and as calm as ever. It is said that this was the last glimpse his devotes had of the Master. He never came out of the river. The tide carried him away and he was gone forever.

With Guru Arjan's martyrdom, the Sikhs' attitude toward life changed. Emulating their Guru, they would readily give their lives for any cause dear to them, whether it was for the protection of the faith, freedom of the country or the integrity of the motherland.

In Guru Arjan we have the culmination of all that Guru Nanak and the three Gurus following him stood for. They combined in themselves the best of Islam and the best of Hinduism. Rather than alienating anyone, they strove for mutual understanding. Venerated equally by the Muslims and the Hindus, they were peace-loving, devoted to meditation, prayer, and service to their fellow man.

Guru Arjan's martyrdom ushered in a new era. It gave a new complexion to the role of the Sikhs in the Punjab. While Guru Arjan's non-violence and martyrdom beautifully reflect the tradition of Guru Nanak, the training that he gave to his successor, Hargobind, was a sign-post of the long drawn-out conflict that followed and that eventually culminated in the momentous turbulence during Guru Gobind Singh's life and times.

3.

The Saint-Soldiers

To a student of Guru Arjan's life, the Guru's martyrdom was an inevitability. The forces of evil and hatred were relentless. Events moved with calamitous certainty. The Guru had attended to all his major assignments. The completion of the Holy Tank called Amritsar and the *Harimandir*, later known as the Golden Temple, attracted Sikh pilgrims from far and near. The town which rose around the Holy Tank grew into a Sikh metropolis. The *Holy Granth* has not only preserved the Holy Word; it has served as a spiritual lighthouse ever since its completion.

Accepting the will of God, Guru Arjan gave up his life, suffering inhuman atrocities in a non-violent manner. Yet the last message he sent to his son was to arm himself fully and prepare for the struggle ahead, which was to be a long drawn-out war against evil and tyranny. The message steeled the heart of his youthful son Hargobind, who had succeeded his father as the sixth Sikh Guru.

It is said, when Bhai Budha, the grand old man of the Sikh brotherhood, brought him *seli*, the sacred headgear of renunciation that Guru Nanak had worn and had bequeathed to his successors one after another, Guru Hargobind put it aside respectfully and asked for a sword instead. Bhai Budha, who had never handled a sword, brought one out and put it on the wrong side. The Guru noticed it and asked for another. "I'll wear two swords," said the Guru, "a sword of *shakti* (power) and a sword of *bhakti* (meditation)."

20

Guru Hargobind combined *piri* (renunciation) and *miri* (royalty). Henceforth the Guru's Sikhs were to carry arms and ride horses. A new concept of the saint-soldier was born.

The Sikhs no longer believed in self-denial alone; they grew increasingly aware of the need for self-assertion as well. Abandoning self-abnegation and renunciation, the Sikhs now wielded arms and lived an active life. They wouldn't frighten anyone, nor were they afraid of anybody. They reared horses, rode on them, and racing and hunting became their pastime. The Guru maintained a regular army. The heroic youth of the nation joined him in large numbers, irrespective of caste and creed. The Sikhs presented the Guru with their best horses and finest weapons as offerings. The Guru built forts and battlements, donned a royal aigrette and was known as *Sacha Padshah,* the True King.

All this was duly reported to King Jehangir who summoned the Guru to Delhi to have a heart-to-heart talk. The Monarch had a guilty conscience on account of Guru Arjan's martyrdom. It is said, the moment Jehangir saw Guru Hargobind, he was completely won over by his youthful charm and spiritual aura. Among other questions, the King asked the Guru which religion was better—Hinduism or Islam. In his reply the Guru quoted from the *Holy Granth:*

> God first created light
> All men are born out of it.
> The whole world emanated from a single spark;
> Who is good and who is bad?
> The Creator is in His creation
> And the creation in the Creator.
> He is everywhere;
> The clay is the same
> The potter fashions models as he fancies.
>
> *(Parbhati—Kabir)*

The King was deeply impressed. He had also been told that the Guru was a great lover of sports. He invited Guru Hargobind to a tiger hunt. The Guru accepted the invitation gladly. It happened that during the chase the King was attacked by a ferocious tiger. The sportsmen accompanying the royal party lost their nerve. Their horses and elephants panicked. The bullets and arrows shot at the tiger missed the target and for a moment it appeared that the beast was going to pounce upon the King. At this moment Guru Hargobind rushed in with his horse, pulled out his sword, and faced the tiger single-handedly. The next instant, the tiger lay slain on the ground. The King was full of gratitude. He admired both the heroic fight and the way the Guru risked his life to save him.

The Emperor became so fond of the Guru that he invited the Guru to accompany him on his next tour of the Kingdom. The Guru's tent was always pitched close to the royal tent. While visiting Agra one day, the King was sitting under a tree. A poor grass-cutter, who had heard about the Guru's visit along with the King, came and, making an offering of a two-paisa coin, pleaded, "You are the True King. I am a poor sinner. Help me wash my sins and attain deliverance from the cycle of life and death." The Monarch heard him and smiled, "The True King is in yonder tent." After saying these words, he directed the grass-cutter to the Guru's tent. Jehangir realized that the True King indeed was one who gave eternal peace and deliverance.

While at Agra, the King was taken seriously ill. The court physicians tried their best but could not cure him. The King decided to consult his astrologers. Chandu Shah, a dignitary who had nursed a grudge against the Guru for not having accepted the hand of his daughter for the Guru's son, conspired with the astrologers. They told the King that his malady was due to an unfavorable conjunction of the stars. It could be remedied if a holy man went to Gwalior Fort and offered continuous prayers to the deity there. Who could be holier than Guru Hargobind, the King's new friend? It was, therefore, decided to ask the Guru to go to Gwalior and undertake penance on behalf of the King. The Guru was aware of Chandu's intrigue; nevertheless, he readily agreed to the proposal and accompanied by an escort of five lieutenants left for Gwalior Fort. The Guru's Sikhs both at Delhi and Amritsar were unhappy to hear about it.

As it happened, a section of Gwalior Fort was used as a prison. The princes detained in the Fort were highly pleased to have the Guru with them. Guru Hargobind found that these princes were in a deplorable plight. He had their living conditions improved. He invited them to join him in morning and evening prayers. In the meantime Chandu wrote to Hari Das, the governor of the Fort, asking him to somehow poison the Guru. Chandu still wanted to be avenged for the indignity he had suffered owing to the Guru's refusal to accept the hand of his daughter. Chandu was not aware that the governor was an ardent devotee of the Guru. Hari Das brought the letter and placed it before Guru Hargobind.

Before long the Monarch fully recovered and the Guru was invited back to the court. But the Guru would not leave the Fort unless the princes detained in the Fort were released. The King would not agree to it. They were either political prisoners or had been detained for default in the payment of large sums of tribute. After a while the King was made to realize that he owed his recovery to the Guru's prayers. It would be the height of ingratitude if he ignored the Guru's request. Therefore, he agreed to the release of the princes. The Guru left the Fort along with fifty-two Hindu princes who had languished in the prison for several years. A part of Gwalior Fort, where the Guru stayed, is still known as *Bandi Chhor,* the liberator of the detained.

When the King met the Guru to thank him, the Guru told the Monarch that his illness was not caused by an unfavorable conjunction of planets. He also explained Chandu's villainy. The King was already aware of Chandu's deceit in plotting to have Guru Arjan tortured to death. In a fit of fury, he handed Chandu over to the Guru as a way to avenge the murder of Guru Arjan.

After a while, Guru Hargobind expressed the desire to return home. When the King heard of this he asked the Guru if he might delay his departure for a few days so that they could travel together. The King wished to spend the summer in Kashmir that year. During the journey, Guru Hargobind's tent was invariably next to the King's. It is said that Nur Jehan, the Queen, took a fancy to the Guru and visited him with her confidante. She was said to be the most charming beauty of her time. The Guru told her that the real charm of a woman was her virtue and her devotion to her husband. Nur Jehan was enchanted to hear the Guru's words.

An old woman named Bhagbhari, who lived in Srinagar, made a fine silk robe with her own hands and longed to present it to the Guru. But the Guru was hundreds of miles away in the Punjab, how would he know about it? The devotee in Bhagbhari, however, was undeterred. The Guru must visit her to receive the gift. Her faith was not disappointed. Before long she had the Guru visiting her. The first thing he came and asked for was the robe that she had completed after years of labor, remembering the Guru every moment.

On his way to Srinagar, Guru Hargobind spent a night with Kattu Shah, a devotee in a village. Hearing that the Divine Master was visiting Kashmir, some of the Sikhs from an out-of-the-way village came to pay homage to him. They too happened to spend a night with Kattu Shah. When he learned that they were carrying a jar of special honey for the Guru, Kattu Shah asked them again and again to let him taste it. The Sikhs who had collected the honey for their Guru would not let Kattu Shah touch the pot, to say nothing of allowing him to taste it. When they arrived in Srinagar and made their offering to the Guru, they discovered much to their embarrassment that the honey had decomposed. It started stinking. The Guru told them that they should not have refused the request of Kattu Shah—the Guru's Sikh—to taste the honey.

About this time Jehangir died and he was succeeded by Shah Jehan. A devotee in Kabul, hearing that the Guru was fond of horses, purchased for him a rare charger. It cost him a lakh of rupees. While crossing the river Attock, the local official noticed the elan of the charger and was fascinated. He felt that he must take possession of the horse for the King. As the Sikh entered Lahore with the prize horse, it was captured by the King's men.

After some time it so happened that the King and the Guru were hunting in the same jungle. Shah Jehan had a rare white hawk presented to him by the King of Iran. Somehow the Guru's party caught hold of the hawk and would not return it. In addition, when the King's men came to collect the hawk, the Sikhs gave them a severe beating and drove them away saying, "We will not return the hawk for the fear of anyone—even the King." The Sikhs wished to avenge themselves for the Mughal soldiers' theft of the charger sent to the Guru by a devotee in Kabul.

How could a King allow it? A few days later when the Guru was busy with preparations for his daughter's marriage, Amritsar was attacked by Mukhlis Khan under the orders of Shah Jehan. This was a challenge that had to be met. Mukhlis Khan, who thought that he would get the King's hawk and the Guru's head by the evening, lost his entire force in the fight. Before long there was another skirmish with Mughal forces at Kartarpur where the royal soldiers were again routed.

One day, while still at Kartarpur, Guru Hargobind went hunting and came across an enchanting spot on the banks of the river Beas. Therefore, the Guru decided to found a new township called Hargobindpur. Before the completion of the town, the Guru made sure that along with the gurdwara, a mosque was also constructed in the town.

The royal hawk was still with the Guru. It became a bone of contention. In the meantime a party of Masands visiting Kabul were bringing along with them Dilbagh and Gulbagh, two rare chargers. These horses could cross a river without the rider getting wet. They were so swift that in a race it seemed as if their hooves never touched the ground. On their way to Amritsar, the horses were seized by the Mughal officials and given over to the Governor. This unfortunate incident led to another fight since the Guru's Sikhs somehow had both the horses retrieved. In this skirmish also, the Mughal forces were mauled and they fled the battlefield in utter disarray.

Painda Khan was one of the most pampered Sardars of Guru Hargobind. He was not only tall and handsome, he was the strongest man in the Guru's army. The Guru was immensely fond of him. He bestowed gifts on him every now and then. Consequently Painda Khan had the best uniform, the best horses and the best treatment. But this seemed to turn his head; he started plotting. He went to the Mughal Court and offered to join the Imperial army. Since he knew all the secrets of the Guru's forces, he received a warm welcome. Painda Khan's strength was legendary. It was said that he could fight an elephant and pulverize a coin with his thumb. Painda Khan told the Mughals that the Guru's army was comprised of the poor and the low castes, the diseased and the disabled; they were weavers and washermen, barbers and ballad-singers.

It was, therefore, decided to send a force under Kale Khan to attack the Guru. Painda Khan was to support the attack. Again a bloody fight raged with heavy carnage. The battle cost the Guru seven hundred of his brave soldiers, while the loss to the Mughal army was heavier, including the killing of Painda Khan, Kale Khan, and several other renowned soldiers.

The Mughal forces immediately withdrew, and the Guru, along with his family and close associates, left for Kiratpur. Budhan Shah, a Muslim divine, had been promised that before he died the Guru would visit him, and the Guru felt that Budhan Shah's end was near. Another factor that probably prevailed with the Guru was the intention to retire to an out-of-the-way, quiet town in order to avoid further bloodshed. Guru Hargobind kept his grandson Har Rai always in his company. Evidently, he was grooming him for the succession.

Guru Hargobind was a tall, handsome man with a fine build and was given to an active life. He was fond of hunting and never avoided a necessary fight. He was a leader of his men and a hero on the battlefield. Like a true soldier, he avoided aggression as far as possible, but when he found himself faced with evil, he struck heavily. He was a fighter for just causes; every time he prevailed in battle. However, due to his sensitive nature the bloodshed and the carnage of the battlefield made him unhappy. Advising his successor that he should keep only 2,200 mounted soldiers for his defense, he bemoaned the loss of many a fine soldier and *Sardar* and passed away contemplating why wars could not be eliminated from the world.

Guru Hargobind's greatest contribution is that he gave a new turn to the Sikh way of life. He turned saints into soldiers and yet remained a man of God. He believed that non-violence is cowardice if it is resorted to out of helplessness or fear. It is the brave and heroic who can be non-violent. Essentially a spiritual leader of a community hardly a hundred years old, he fought a number of battles with the Imperial forces and every time vanquished his foe because the truth was always on his side. It was always a fight in self-defense and never a war of aggression. This new trend that he gave to Sikh polity ultimately found its finest expression in his grandson Guru Gobind Singh, the tenth Sikh Guru.

Guru Har Rai was just 14 years old when he became the seventh Sikh Guru. In fact, he was nominated for succession because his father Bhai Gurditta had died an untimely death. He was Guru Hargobind's eldest son.

Guru Hargobind detested miracle-making. He felt that it was interfering with the ways of God. Baba Atal, another of the Guru's sons, had a playmate who was bitten by a snake and died. Baba Atal could not believe it and in all his innocence approached the dead body and said, "Mohan, get up, you owe me a turn in the game." It is said that the dead youth opened his eyes at the call and walked off to play with his companion! When Guru Hargobind heard about it, he was distressed. "How can anyone interfere with the ways of God?" he asked. Baba Atal heard the reprimand and took it to heart. Sitting by the side of Kaulsar, he said his prayers and gave his life for the life he had saved.

When Shah Jehan heard about Guru Har Rai's succession, he too realized that it was best to make friends with this heroic and self-respecting community. Accordingly, when his son Dara Shikoh fell seriously ill, he approached the Guru for his blessings and the young prince is said to have been cured with an herb Guru Har Rai sent to Delhi.

But this amity with the Delhi Darbar was short-lived. Aurangzeb, the third son of King Shah Jehan, usurped the throne and chased away Dara Shikoh, his eldest brother. While in flight, Dara Shikoh met Guru Har Rai. According to the tradition of the

Guru's household, Guru Har Rai received the prince with due courtesy and gave him all the help that he needed. Dara Shikoh, who was a scholar and a God-fearing man, told the Guru that he was not at all interested in the Delhi throne and that he would be happier if he were left alone for spiritual pursuits. However, Aurangzeb captured Dara Shikoh and executed him after having him condemned by the *qazi* for deviating from the Islamic creed.

After Aurangzeb was firmly settled on the Mughal throne, he turned his attention to the Sikhs. An excuse was readily available. The Guru had met and blessed Dara Shikoh, an enemy of the King.

Guru Har Rai passed away at the early age of thirty in 1661. Though the records are silent about it, the end must have come unexpectedly, probably owing to some fatal illness. But just before his death, he had his second son Harkrishan ordained as the Guru. The stewardship of Guru Har Rai and Guru Harkrishan was a sort of interregnum in the life of the Sikh community, before it began a new path of no compromise with injustice and evil.

Guru Tegh Bahadur, who succeeded Guru Harkrishan, was essentially contemplative by temperament. But the conditions in the Punjab and the rest of the country would not allow him a peaceful life.

Though God-fearing and pious, Aurangzeb honestly believed that Hinduism was utterly misconceived, decadent, and idolatrous. It was for their own good if he could rid his people of superstitious and anti-God practices.

Another factor that contributed to Aurangzeb's ill-conceived adventure was his anxiety to improve his own image. He had imprisoned his father and starved him to death. He had his brothers Dara Shikoh and Murad murdered. He grievously insulted his son Muazzim, who later on ascended the throne as Bahadur Shah. Aurangzeb was poorly regarded in the Islamic world, and he wished to secure a berth for himself in the next world. He therefore decided to turn the country into Dar-ul-Islam, the abode of Muslims, and issued instructions to his Governors to launch a mass conversion drive of the Hindus.

In Kashmir, the Governor realized that the Hindus had started fleeing his province. If this continued, he felt, he would be left with hardly anyone to rule over. He therefore invited the leading brahmins of the community for a dialogue. He explained to them his helplessness in view of the firm orders from Delhi. After protracted discussion it was decided that the Hindu community should be given six months to make up its mind.

Kashmiri brahmins decided to make a pilgrimage to Amarnath and seek intervention of the deity. It is said that while at the Amarnath temple, a member of the group of worshipers, Pandit Kirpa Ram, dreamt that they could be protected only by Guru Tegh Bahadur, the ninth in succession to Guru Nanak, who was the savior in the Kaliyuga. Immediately they left for the Punjab and reached Anandpur. They lost no time in explaining their predicament to the Guru. The Guru heard their tale of woe and was lost in deep contemplation when Gobind, his young son walked in. "What is bothering you, dear father?" he asked. The Guru explained to him the situation. "They can be saved only if a great soul can offer himself for martyrdom." "Then who is greater than you?" remarked the future saint-soldier of the Sikhs. The father was assured that Gobind was ready to take over. He advised the visiting supplicators to go back and inform their tormentors that they would be willing to accept Islam if Guru Tegh Bahadur could first be persuaded to do so.

The Guru was summoned to Delhi and put in jail. "If you are a man of God, you must work a miracle," the King said. The Guru would not purchase his release the way a juggler earns his living. Then the inevitable took place. The *qazi* gave his *fatwa* and the Guru was executed. Thus, while Guru Nanak refused to wear the sacred thread, Guru Tegh Bahadur gave his life so that the right of a community to wear the sacred thread and practice its faith was protected. This makes Guru Tegh Bahadur's martyrdom unique in history. People give their lives for principles dear to them, ideals cherished by them and faiths they hold. There is hardly anyone who has staked his life for other people's faith. The supreme sacrifice made by Guru Tegh Bahadur stemmed the tide of intolerance in the sub-continent and inculcated in the people respect for other religions.

4.

Birth of the Khalsa

Guru Tegh Bahadur's public execution in Delhi outraged the conscience of the entire Sikh brotherhood. After Guru Arjan Dev's martyrdom in Lahore, the slaughtering of another peace-loving, non-violent man of God such as Guru Tegh Bahadur gave a rude shock to the young community. The Sikhs streamed towards Anandpur from near and far to be with the young Guru.

Born in Patna in 1666 and brought up for the grim struggle ahead, the young Gobind Rai, rather than being overwhelmed with his tragic loss, evinced firm determination and tenacity of will to fight the forces of evil and bigotry in defense of the poor and the *dharma*. The disconsolate Sikhs who flocked to Anandpur saw in their Guru the promised savior and the man of the hour.

A soldier of destiny, the tenth Guru started consolidating his resources and preparing himself and his people for the gruesome fight until the poison that had permeated the body politic of the country had been completely rooted out. Guru Gobind realized the need to give Sikhism a distinct identity. Islam under rulers like Aurangzeb had become rigid, narrow-minded, and uncompromising, and Hinduism had been enfeebled by ritualism.

As a first step, it was necessary to consolidate resources and manpower, which necessitated a discreet pause during which links were forged with Sikhs spread all over India and abroad, including Kabul, Kandahar, Bulkh, and Bokhara.

The Guru was visited by his followers who brought him highly precious gifts. Duni Chand, a Sikh from Kabul, brought a canopy that was worth two and a half lakhs of rupees. During his visit to Assam, Guru Tegh Bahadur had blessed a ruler who was issueless. As a result, a son was born to the ruler. While the raja had died, the queen came with the prince, called Ratan Lal, to pay homage to the Guru with various gifts, including an elephant of uncanny intelligence who carried out various commands to the delight of the spectators. He washed the Guru's feet with water and then wiped them with a towel. He fetched arrows discharged by the guru. At night he showed the way with lighted candles held in this trunk. He performed other feats as well.

The Guru practiced archery, went out on *shikar,* and played mock battles with his companions. He had a huge drum made and collected his people, whenever he required them, by beating the drum.

The Guru also devoted himself to research, literary, and artistic activity. He had fifty-two eminent poets working with him; poetic symposia were held frequently. The Guru, who was a scholar of Sanskrit and Persian, participated in them. His writings are a clear break with the tradition of his predecessors. He wrote powerful verse which is replete with images of war and warriors from ancient mythology and folklore. He worshipped God; he also had an unmistakable love of the sword.

The Guru had four sons—Ajit Singh, Jujhar Singh, Zorawar Singh, and Fateh Singh. He trained them to ride horses, handle arms, and to read and interpret classics. The Guru also engaged scholars to translate philosophical treatises from Sanskrit into the popular language of the common people.

For the Baisakhi fair in 1699, the Guru issued a general invitation to his Sikhs throughout the length and breadth of the country to visit Anandpur. He advised Sikhs to come with unshorn hair. Several thousand Sikhs came to participate in the fair in response to the Guru's call.

On the morning of the main fair day after the hymn-singing had concluded, the Guru appeared on the dais with an unsheathed sword dazzling in his hand and asked the audience, "My sword is thirsty. It needs the blood of a Sikh to quench its thirst. Is there anyone in the audience who is willing to offer his head?" There was consternation among all those present.

"Is there no one who is willing to present his head to satisfy my sword?" the Guru repeated.

The gathering grew more uneasy. "Do I understand that there is none among my Sikhs who is willing to sacrifice his life for his Guru?" As the Guru repeated his call the third time, a Sikh called Daya Ram, a Khatri from Lahore, thirty years old, rose from the crowd to offer his head. "It's yours in life and death," said the Sikh humbly. The Guru caught hold of him by his arm and led him to a tent pitched adjacent to the dais. There was a thud of the sword.

A moment later the Guru appeared, with his sword dripping with blood. "I want another head," shouted the Guru. There was panic in the audience. They even doubted if their leader was sane at all. Still, before the guru could repeat his call, another Sikh, this time a Jat from Haryana, rose and placed his head at the disposal of his Master. The Guru pulled him into the tent, in a strange frenzy. Again there was the thud of the sword followed by a stream of blood flowing out of the tent. And as before, the Guru came out of the tent with blood dripping from his sharp-edged sword.

"I want another head, the third." He stood glowing with fiery eyes. Even at his first call, Mohkam Chand, a Sikh from far-off Dwarka, hurried to the scaffolding, apologizing for not offering himself earlier. The same frightful thud of the sword followed; and the red blood squirted out of the sacrificial tent. The thirst of the Guru's sword was still not quenched. He came out the fourth time demanding yet another head. The blade of his sword was stained with blood. Some people from the hysterical crowd started running away. "I want the fourth head." The Guru looked around and before he finished making this call, Himmat Chand, who had come all the way from Jagannathpuri in Orissa, rushed to the Guru. His head was at his Master's disposal. Like the other three Sikhs, he was also led to the tent. The thud of the sword was repeated and the stream of blood flowing from the tent was augmented with fresh blood. With blood dripping once again, the Guru asked for yet another head. By now, the gathering had thinned considerably. Sahib Chand of Bidar rushed to the dais and fell at the Guru's feet for not responding to his call all the while. The Guru led the fifth Sikh also into the tent.

Terror-stricken, some Sikhs ran to inform the Guru's mother; others thought of seeking the intervention of the Guru's senior advisers. They had gathered to celebrate the festival of Baisakhi and the Guru had started butchering them. They were on the horns of a dilemma. They did not know what to do, when suddenly from behind the tent, they saw the five faithful Sikhs emerge one after another, radiant and beaming, like five resplendent stars descended from heaven! They were followed by the Guru glowing with a new confidence. The audience burst into spontaneous joy. They hailed the Guru with slogans: "The Guru is great!" "Long live the Guru!" "Glory to the Guru!" Shouting such slogans, they were jumping with joy when the Guru raised his hand and silenced them. "Great are the Five Faithful! Glory to them! They are the chosen ones. They have found immortality. Those who know how to die, only they win deliverance from the cycle of life and death," said the Guru.

The Guru, it is said, had slaughtered only goats. Every time he took a Sikh inside the tent, he slaughtered a goat and came out with its blood dripping from the blade of his sword.

The Guru then had a steel vessel brought and poured water into it. The Five Faithful Sikhs were asked to recite hymns from the sacred scriptures turn by turn, while the Guru stirred the water with a double-edged dagger called *khanda*. The Guru was preparing *amrit*—nectar to baptize Guru Nanak's Sikhs, to bestow on them the name of Khalsa, the chosen ones. As the Five Faithful Sikhs were reciting the Holy Word, clad in their blue robes of divine angels, Mata Sahib Devan came with *patashas*—sugar-candy—as an offering. The Guru was most happy. "It is a timely gift," he said and, taking the *patashas*, put them into the vessel. "It is marrying valor with compassion," said the Guru. "The dagger was to turn the Sikhs into heroes, the sugarcandy will foster in them the milk of human kindness.''

When the recitation from the pre-determined text of the scripture was over, the Guru blessed the five beloved faithful with the nectar, the draught of immortality and knowledge sublime.

After the Sikhs had been thus blessed, the Guru himself stood before them with his hands folded and prayed to the Five Faithful to baptize him in return. Thus the Guru turned himself into a disciple. It was the first time in the annals of history that the Master sat at the feet of his disciples asking them to be blessed with a draught of nectar. The moment he had the sublime sip, he then became known as Guru Gobind Singh. The Five Faithful Sikhs and thousands of the Guru's devotees who had gathered at Anandpur were also blessed with the nectar and called *singhs* (*singh* means lion). According to the report of a diarist of the Mughal court to the Emperor in Delhi, 20,000 Sikhs were anointed on that blessed Baisakhi day. This was the birth of the Khalsa, the reincarnation of Guru Nanak's Sikhs. A draught of *amrit* and every Sikh became a Singh, a lion. Everyone had to sip *amrit* from a common vessel, thereby joining the eternal brotherhood and casting away the barriers of caste and creed.

The Guru then enjoined those who had been blessed with *amrit* to wear long hair *(kesh)*. The hair is sacred. It is the symbol of the Khalsa, the pure. They were also to wear a steel bangle *(kada)* on their wrist. It should serve as a reminder of their commitment to truth. An anointed Sikh must also wear short pants *(kachha)* to ensure cleanliness. The Sikh should have a comb *(kangha)* in the hair to keep it tidy. Also he should always carry a dagger *(kirpan)* as a weapon of defense.

The Guru was aware that the need of the hour was an army of saint-soldiers who could effectively fight the forces of evil, exploitation of the poor, and communal hatred in Indian society.

The anointed Sikh was not to smoke or take any other intoxicants. He must be loyal to his spouse and not covet other women. All Sikhs were equal; there was no high or low caste among the Khalsa. The Khalsa believed in one God, said his prescribed prayers daily, and did not worship idols or images. The Khalsa must help the needy and protect the poor. The Sikhs who adopt the prescribed way of life are as good as the Guru. The Guru is the Khalsa and the Khalsa is the Guru.

After the grand baptism, the Guru declared that all his Sikhs were to be known as Singhs (lions). The baptism had turned jackals into lions. The Khalsa must fight oppression. It is maintained that having been anointed with *amrit*, a single Sikh could fight a lakh and a quarter enemies.

And indeed, the Sikhs did do this miracle. They fought fourteen times against the well-disciplined imperial army—fourteen pitched battles—and not less than twelve times they defeated the enemy, and made him withdraw, miserably mauled and routed.

Fighting against evil and injustice, Guru Gobind Singh suffered grievous losses personally. His father was martyred. His mother died in captivity. Two of his sons met their end fighting single-handedly against heavy odds. Their father watched them from a battlement besieged by a rabid host. His two younger sons were walled in alive. Hundreds of his loyal lieutenants and thousands of his faithful followers gave their lives fighting for their Guru. His prize horses and precious manuscripts were lost. There came a time when he was left all alone, without a horse, without any arms, with no attendant. Having wandered through hostile jungles, his clothes were torn. Walking day and night, his shoes were worn out. With thorns pricking his feet, lonely and forlorn, it is said, he reached Machhiwada jungle. He lay down on the bare earth with a stone for his pillow. It was here that he sang what is now regarded as one of his most famous hymns:

> Go tell the plight of His devotees
>   to my beloved Lord.
> The luxury of soft beds is agony without Him;
> It's like living in a snake-pit,
> The goblet is poison and the cup a dagger,
> Life is like receiving a butcher's punches.

I would rather live in hiding, with my beloved.
It's hell living with strangers without Him.

He who lived like a prince in royal splendor was rendered
homeless. He was being chased by the enemy forces from town to
town, from wilderness to wilderness. Even then he was not
demoralized. While camping at village Dinga, the Guru wrote a
letter to Aurangzeb in response to his invitation to see him. The
Guru's letter is known as *Zafar Nama*, the Epistle of Victory.

The guru told the King that he had taken up arms because he
had exhausted all other means of redress. The Guru continued:

"If I had not believed your word and your oath on the
Quran, I wouldn't have left my town. If I had known that you
are deceitful and crafty like a fox, I wouldn't have been here
today . . .

"Every soldier of your army who left his defenses to attack
us was slaughtered. . . . Many were done to death on either
side with arrows and bullets showered on them. The whole
earth was smeared with red blood. Heads and legs lay in heaps.
The arrows whizzed and bows twanged, the clamor all over
reached heavens. My heroic soldiers fought like lions. But how
could forty men, even the bravest soldiers, succeed against
countless odds?

"You are faithless and irreligious. You neither know God
nor Muhammad. A religious man never breaks his promise.
Had the prophet been here, I would make it a point to tell him
about your treachery.

"What if my four sons have been killed, I live to take their
revenge. It's no heroism to extinguish a few sparks. You have
only excited a devastating fire.

"You have the pride of your empire, while I am proud of
the Kingdom of God. You must not forget that this world is
like a caravanserai and one must leave it sooner or later. . . ."

The King received the Guru's letter and was struck with

remorse. He removed all restrictions on the movements of the Guru and gave orders that Guru Gobind Singh and his Sikhs should be harassed no longer. Aurangzeb's conscience seemed to prick him for the cruelties inflicted on the Guru and his Sikhs. It is said that he then took to his bed and soon thereafter he died.

After Aurangzeb's proclamation, the Guru came to Talwandi Sabo, now known as Damdama Sahib. The local chief called Dalla came to him and offered condolences on the martyrdom of his four sons. Dalla led a contingent of four hundred men and said again and again that if he had known it, he would have placed his men at the Guru's disposal. "Each one of them would have died fighting for you." As he was talking in this vein, a Sikh came and presented a gun to the Guru. The Guru asked Dalla to go and get one of his men so that he could check his aim with the new weapon. Dalla was flabbergasted to hear it. But when the Guru insisted, he went over to his people and as he feared, not one of his men came forward to serve as the Guru's target. Dalla was greatly mortified. He returned to the Guru, his head hanging in shame.

The moment the Guru saw him, he asked one of his attendants to go and tell the two young Sikhs tying their turbans at a little distance, that the Guru wanted one of them to serve as his target to test the new gun that he had been presented with. As the young Sikhs heard it, they came running to the Guru. Both of them vied with each other for the honor. They happened to be brothers. The elder brother said that he has a better claim to serve his father, the Guru, while the younger one said he must have his share of the father's property. Dalla was astonished to see this devotion. The Guru told him that it was *amrit* which made such heroes of men. It made sparrows challenge hawks.

It was at Damdama Sahib that the Guru's consort joined him after the battle. It is said that when she arrived, the Guru was in a congregation. "Where are my children, my four darling sons?" the bereaved mother cried in agony.

"Here are thousands of them, all your children," the Guru told her, pointing to the congregation.

It was again at Damdama Sahib that Guru Gobind Singh

found time to redictate the *Holy Granth*, incorporating into it Guru Tegh Bahadur's hymns.

After Aurangzeb's death, there was the usual scramble for succession to the Mughal throne. Aurangzeb's eldest son Bahadur Shah was in Peshawar, therefore his younger brother Azam proclaimed himself King. Bahadur Shah sought the Guru's assistance. Since he was the rightful successor, the Guru was keen to ensure that like his father, Bahadur Shah was not misled. He placed a detachment at his disposal. Bahadur Shah was victorious and invited the Guru for his coronation where he presented him with a robe of honor and several precious gifts.

They became such good friends that Bahadur Shah persuaded the Guru to accompany him to the South on his tour. It was indeed a victory of truth over falsehood, a vindication of good-neighborliness and communal amity over bigotry and narrow parochialism.

5.

The Word Became the Guru

The compilation and the consecration of the *Holy Granth* is a fascinating story of catholicity of viewpoint, brotherhood of man, and communal amity.

Says Guru Nanak:

What I am communicated by my Master
I transmit unto you.

The Guru himself was only the medium; the Holy spirit is said to have traveled from Guru Nanak through the rest of the nine Sikh Gurus succeeding him, until it reached Guru Gobind Singh, the "tenth Guru Nanak," who said:

As ordained by the Lord Eternal
A new way of life is evolved;
All the Sikhs are asked
To accept the *Holy Granth* as the Guru.
Guru Granth should be accepted
As the living Guru.
Those who wish to meet God
Will find him in the Word.

Thus the Word became the Guru. The stewardship of the *Sikh*

Panth—the Sikh way of life—was entrusted to the *Holy Granth*. Guru Gobind Singh declared unequivocally that those who wished to seek God would find him in the Scripture. With the passing away of Guru Gobind Singh, the tradition of the Guru in the form of physical being came to an end. The *Holy Granth* was consecrated as the Guru. Those who looked for His blessings found them in the Book.

The Sikhs came to give the same esteem, the same veneration to the *Holy Granth* as to the living Guru. They prostrate before it the first thing every morning, make offerings of all sorts, and seek guidance from the Scripture by reading, reciting, and singing hymns.

And the text does not belong to the Sikh Gurus alone. The *Holy Granth* has, aside from the hymns of the Sikh Gurus, compositions of thirty-six great sages belonging to the various castes and creeds, religions and avocations. Among them are Jaidev of Bengal; Gurdas of Awadh; Namdev, Trilochan, and Parmanand of Maharashtra; Beni, Ramanand, Pipa, Sain, Kabir, Ravidas, and Bhikan of Uttar Pradesh; Dhanna of Rajasthan and Farid of Multan in the Punjab. Not only this, but some of them even belonged to the so-called lowest of the low castes. Kabir was a weaver, Sadhna a butcher, Namdev a seamster, Sain a barber, and Ravidas a tanner. The compiler of the *Holy Granth* did not allow communal or religious distinctions to come in its way. Dhanna was a Jat, while Pipa was a king. Farid was a Muslim divine and Bhikka a learned scholar of Islam, while Jaidev was a Hindu mystic and poet.

Thus, when a Sikh bows before and seeks guidance from the *Holy Granth*, he offers his devotion as much to Farid, the renowned Muslim saint, and Jaidev, a Hindu *bhakta* of Krishna, as to Guru Nanak or Guru Arjan, the compiler of the *Granth*. It is a commonwealth of the experience of the enlightened ones.

Be that as it may, it is said that some of the Guru's detractors made a complaint to the Mughal Emperor Akbar that the work compiled by Guru Arjan Dev included compositions that maligned Islam and Hinduism. Akbar happened to be touring the Punjab in

those days. He summoned the Guru along with the manuscript of
the *Holy Granth.* While the guru did not consider it necessary to go
personally, he sent two of his trusted lieutenants with the compilation. It is said the King had a hymn read to him at random. It
was a composition of Guru Arjan himself:

> From clay and light God created the world;
> The sky, the earth, trees, and water
>   are made by Him.
>
> * * * * *
>
> One must restrain oneself,
> Hell is the punishment of the defaulter;
> The miracle man, the riches, brothers,
>   courtiers, kingdom, and palaces;
> None will come to your rescue at the hour
>   of final departure.

The King heard the hymn and was deeply impressed. However,
the detractors contended that the Emperor was intentionally read a
piece that was not objectionable. At this, the King himself pointed
out a hymn and had it read to him. This too was found inoffensive.
At this the wicked contended that since none of them knew the
Gurmukhi script, the Guru's agent read the hymns from memory
rather than the text indicated. Akbar now had Sahib Dyal, a local
citizen, sent for to read aloud a piece pointed out to him by the
King. The hymn read was:

> You don't see God who dwells in your heart,
> And you carry about an idol on your neck.
> A non-believer, you wander about churning water,
> And you die harassed in delusion.
> The idol you call God will drown with you.

The Emperor heard it and was greatly moved. He said it was a
work worthy of reverence. He made his offering of thirty-one gold
mohurs to the *Holy Granth,* complimented Guru Arjan on the

compilation, and promised to visit Amritsar personally in the near future to pay his homage to the Guru. The Emperor remembered to keep his promise.

The compilation of the *Holy Granth* was preceded by an unhappy family dispute. Guru Angad, who followed Guru Nanak, was not his son. He was one of the disciples who was considered fittest for the honor. Similarly, Guru Amar Das, the third Guru, was also a devotee of Guru Angad and no blood relative as such. Accordingly, when the time came to name his successor, Guru Amar Das decided in favor of Guru Ram Das, in preference to his two sons, Mohan and Mohri.

Guru Ram Das selected one of his younger sons, Guru Arjan, to be his successor. This offended his eldest who had expected to be named Guru. The eldest son started maligning Guru Arjan and began to present himself as the Guru. It was he who had complained to the Emperor against the *Holy Granth*. It was also learned that Prithi Chand had started composing his own verses and passing them on to the Sikhs as scripture. When Guru Arjan became aware of this, he decided to compile the compositions of Guru Nanak and his successors in an authentic volume to insulate them against any spurious interpolations.

Once the decision was made, Guru Arjan went about this ambitious project in a systematic manner. As a first step, he sent scribes to the various places visited by Guru Nanak and his successors to contact those whom the Gurus had met, and obtain from them the authentic versions of the hymns. A Sikh was even sent as far away as Sri Lanka. When it was reported that Mohan, the eldest son of Guru Amar Das, would not part with the hymns in his custody, Guru Arjan called on him personally at Goindwal and persuaded him to cooperate in the noble undertaking. On the way back Guru Arjan also visited Datu, Guru Angad's son, and collected whatever manuscripts were available from him.

In view of the importance of the task, Guru Arjan had a special library set up in a quiet corner of Ramsar, one of the holy tanks in Amritsar. Bhai Gurdas, the eminent Sikh author, was entrusted with the job of preparing the master-copy. Guru Arjan himself dictated the text. When the *Holy Granth* was ready, it was installed with due ceremony at the *Harimandir* and Bhai Budha, the oldest living disciple of Guru Nanak, was appointed the first custodian. As a token of appreciation, Guru Arjan offered to include the compositions of Bhai Gurdas in the *Holy Granth,* but because of his modesty, he denied himself the great honor.

The *Holy Granth* was redictated by Guru Gobind Singh, the tenth and last living Sikh Guru, towards the close of his life. He had Guru Tegh Bahadur's compositions incorporated in the body of the text. However, Guru Gobind Singh's modesty did not allow him to include his own verse in it.

But Guru Gobind Singh does have a massive volume of compositions to his credit. Maybe the consideration that weighed against the inclusion of his own verse was that the compilation as done by Guru Arjan would get too unwieldy.

The hymns compiled in the *Holy Granth* have been arranged in various *ragas* according to Hindustani music. The hymns under every musical measure are led by Guru Nanak and other Sikh Gurus in chronological order, the compositions of the *bhaktas* following them. There are approximately 6,000 hymns in the *Holy Granth* in thirty-one *ragas.*

It is said that Kahna, Chhajju, Pilu, and a few other contemporary poets approached Guru Arjan and offered their verses for inclusion in the *Holy Granth.* The Guru duly considered their compositions, but regretted his inability to include them in the volume for one reason or another.

Some of the bards who subscribed to the Sikh faith and composed several panegyrics in praise of the Sikh Gurus requested the incorporation of their compositions. A few of these were included in the *Holy Granth.*

The scripting of the text was completed in 1604, Guru Arjan providing the epilogue:

Three things are there in the vessel
Truth, contentment, and learning.
The ambrosial Name of God is added to it,

The name that is everybody's sustenance.
He who eats and enjoys it
Shall be saved.
One must not abandon this gift,
It should ever remain dear to one's heart.
The dark ocean of the world
Can be crossed by clinging to His feet,
Nanak, it is He who is everywhere.

(Mundawani)

This was followed by an apologia in utmost modesty:

I can't measure Your grace
You've made me worthy of You.
I am full of blemishes;
I have no virtue
You have been compassionate.
Compassionate You have been and kind.
Thus I met the true Guru.
Says Nanak, I live on the Name alone,
It pleases my heart and soul.

(Mundawani)

The *raga mala* following this, however, does not tally with the *ragas* in the *Holy Granth,* and its inclusion has been a subject of controversy for a long time.

The text in the *Holy Granth* had the utmost sanctity accorded to it since its compilation. Not even the change of a single syllable has been permitted. For a long time, the Sikhs would not permit the words in the text to be written or printed separately; they continued to be copied as a continuous text following the original done by Bhai Gurdas.

It is said that on one occasion Aurangzeb took exception to a particular verse in the *Holy Granth*. Ram Rai, the son of Guru Har Rai, the seventh Sikh Guru, who was staying with Aurangzeb as his guest, altered the original slightly to please the King. When it was reported to the Guru, he was mortified and sent word to his son never to show his face to him again.

Once Guru Har Rai was resting. A Sikh entered his room while reciting hymns from the *Holy Granth*. The moment the Guru heard him, he rose and sat upright in reverence to the Holy Word.

The *Holy Granth* is the most ambitious compilation of devotional verse. It is also the most representative of its times. It has a grand design and a highly scientific manner of presentation. The pattern adopted by Guru Arjan was designed to permit the incorporation of later compositions without interfering with the text of the works already compiled. For example, Guru Gobind Singh didn't have to disturb the arrangement when he added Guru Tegh Bahadur's compositions:

The *Holy Granth* opens with the *mul mantra,* or basic postulate:

There is but one God
His Name is Truth
He is the Creator
He fears none nor does he hate anyone
He is in the image of the Eternal
He is beyond birth and death
He is self-existent
He can be attained by the Guru's grace.

The thirty-one *ragas* included in the *Holy Granth* are: Sri Rag, Majh, Gauri, Asa, Gujri, Dev Gandhari, Bihagda Wadhans, Sorath, Dhanasri, Jaitsri, Todi, Bairadi, Tilang, Suhi, Bilawal, Gaud, Ramkali, Nat Narayan, Mali Gauda, Maru, Tukhari, Kidar, Bhairav, Basant, Sarang, Malhar, Kanada, Kalyan, Prabhati, and Jaijaivanti. Following the compositions figuring under the various *ragas,* there are a number of other hymns like Sanskrit *slokas,* the *Gatha,* and the *Swaiyyas.*

The order of hymns usually followed under each *raga* is as follows: *Shabad, Ashtapadis, Chhand, Var* and hymns contributed by the *bhaktas.* In order to guard against the risk of interpolations, every Shabad and every verse in the *Holy Granth* is numbered and recorded. The numbering also makes it more convenient to locate the hymns.

As a literary work, the *Holy Granth* has many sections of excellent poetry from the viewpoint of both form and content. The language varies from Sanskrit to Persian, to various dialects of Punjabi. The poetic forms are as varied as they are original. They invariably reflect the mood of the text and succeed eminently in communicating it to the reader. The Gurus and the *bhaktas* take ample liberties with the form and do not seem to observe the rigidities of traditional poetic molds. In order that their compositions should be popular, the Gurus preferred the measure and tunes of the folk ballads and folk-songs. This must have helped the Sikhs to sing the hymns to their proper tunes. It is a great pity that since Hindustani music has an oral tradition, most of the tunes prescribed by the respective authors have been lost over time.

The poetry of the *Holy Granth* is a gold mine of philosophic thought. It is highly revealing and reflects a way of life which is as simple as it is ennobling. Every word of the *Holy Granth* inspires and elevates. It has appeal equally to the erudite scholar and the least literate reader. It evokes veneration as much from the Sikhs as from the Hindus and Muslims alike.

It must, however, be understood that paper and the printed word are not the Guru. They are only the vehicle. The Guru is what is contained within the text, what one imbibes by reading the text, the revelation, the vision, the ecstasy. However, the fact remains that while the container that holds the nectar may not be nectar itself, it is no commonplace container.

Sikhism
in Modern India

6.
Maharaja Ranjit Singh's Secularism

It is difficult to define secularism. Secularism does not just pertain to worldly things, or just to things that are not particularly religious, spiritual or sacred. Instead it is a wedding between reason and faith. Secularism is religious neutralism on the part of the State that decides issues on merit, irrespective of considerations of caste, creed or color.

According to this concept of the term, Maharaja Ranjit Singh's regime was truly secular. Built on the ruins of the Mughal Empire, his kingdom extended from Tibet to Sind and from Kabul to the Sutlej. It is said that eighty percent of the population of the territory he ruled over was Muslim, ten percent Hindu and the remaining ten percent were his co-religionists.

He was a devout Sikh. Every day he said his prayers after an early morning bath, and paid his homage to the *Holy Granth*. Such was his faith in the Sikh scriptures that he never launched any expedition or project, or undertook even a trivial matter, without seeking guidance from the Book. It is said that he respectfully carried a copy of the *Holy Granth* even on the battlefield on an elephant especially designated for that purpose. Once he was found guilty of a lapse as a Gursikh. He presented himself at Akal Takht, the highest Sikh religious seat, and surrendered himself for punishment to atone for it. The Maharaja received lashes on his bare back served by Akali Phula Singh.

He never discriminated against any other faith. Once he told his Foreign Minister, Fakir Azizuddin, "God intended my looking upon all the religions with one eye, that is why I was deprived of the other eye."

Born in November 1780 at his maternal grandparents' house, he was given the name of Budh Singh—the man of learning. However, when the news was communicated to his father, Maha Singh Sakarchakya, who was at the time engaged in a skirmish with a neighboring chief, he changed his son's name to Ranjit Singh—the man of victory. Ranjit Singh won many a battle, but remained unlettered all his life.

It was not until he was seventeen that he became the real master of his estate. He consolidated his position through matrimonial alliances with Kanhyas by marrying Mahtab Kaur, the daughter of Sada Kaur (whose husband had been killed by Ranjit Singh's father) and Raj Kaur, a sister of Nakkai Sardar. For obvious reasons, it was a strange love-hate relation that he developed with Sada Kaur, his mother-in-law. It helped and hindered his adventures for years to come. It is amazing that, even at that early age, Ranjit Singh made important moves towards consolidating the Sikh Sardars in the Punjab who were broken up into twelve principalities called *misals*.

A welcome opportunity came his way when Shah Zaman cast his "owl-like shadow over the Punjab." Under Ranjit Singh's leadership the Sikh fraternity met at Akal Takht. This meeting was called *Sarbat Khalsa*. Because the meeting was held at a holy spot in Amritsar, all decisions undertaken had religious sanction. A number of Sardars were in favor of fleeing to the hills as they had done earlier, but Ranjit Singh remained adamant. It was eventually decided to give fight to the intruder under Ranjit Singh's command. Under his inspiring leadership, the Sikhs not only drove Shah Zaman back, but a time came when Ranjit Singh climbed the Musummum Burj in Lahore Fort, where the invader was holding court, and shouted, "O you progeny of Abdali, come out and measure your sword with the progeny of Charhat Singh." It is said that the Afghan soldiers became afraid of the Sikhs. They would not stir out of their barracks at night. Ranjit Singh ultimately chased Shah Zaman up to the banks of the river Indus, inflicting grievous losses on the enemy. Thus, the belief that grass never grows where the Afghan horses tread was belied for good.

After the retreat of the Afghans, Lahore was occupied by three Sardars of whom Chet Singh was the most impetuous. They misruled the town, indulging in drinking and debauchery. The people got sick of them and Muslims and non-Muslims alike sent word to Ranjit Singh to come and take over the town. When Ranjit Singh heard about the state of affairs, he sent his trusted lieutenant, Abdul Rehman, to verify the truth of this story. After he was reassured, Ranjit Singh marched at the head of 25,000 troops and occupied Lahore, the biggest and most prestigious town of the Punjab, without any bloodshed. After taking over the town, the first thing Ranjit Singh did was to go and pay homage to the *Badshahi Masjid*—the Royal Mosque.

Ranjit Singh paid immediate attention to the administration of the town and welfare of the people. No one was allowed to practice highhandedness or oppression. Even if the Maharaja himself issued an unfair order it could be brought to his notice for review. The judges were asked to administer justice in accordance with the *Shastras* and the *Quran*. Nizamuddin was appointed Chief *Qazi*. He had Mohammed Shahpuri and Saidullah as his *muftis*. There was a chain of *Yunani* dispensaries in the town under Hakim Nuruddin, who was the Chief Medical Officer; Imam Baksh was appointed *Kotwal* of Lahore.

Maharaja Ranjit Singh had several high positions in his army entrusted to Hindus and Muslims. There were more than forty high-ranking Muslim officers in his forces. At least two of them were generals.

After Ranjit Singh had captured a chain of small states around Lahore, he sent a force of 20,000 men led by Misr Diwan Chand, a Hindu general, to attack Multan. He was to be assisted by Ilahi Bakhsh, a Muslim general of repute. It was a keenly fought battle. Nawab Muzaffar Khan of Multan fought to the last. But ultimately, victory fell into the hands of the Maharaja's forces. This conquest also helped subdue a number of Muslim states like Bahawalpur, Dera Ghazi Kahn, Dera Ismail Khan, and Mankera. Immediately after the victory at Multan, the Maharaja went to the mausoleum of Shah Abdul Mali built by Mian Ghausa, one of Ranjit Singh's commanders, who was killed in the fighting, to pay homage at the shrine.

Then followed a series of important conquests at Jammu, Srinagar, Peshawar, and Kabul. It was a practice of the Maharaja to endow all the dispossessed chiefs with *jagirs* and as far as possible establish permanent friendships with them. He was particularly considerate towards the Muslim rulers.

The Maharaja handled the English imperialists with great tact and as long as he lived, he kept them at arm's length. He employed foreigners to modernize his army and administration. It is said that there were thirty-seven foreigners in his service. They included three Englishmen, twelve Frenchmen, four Italians, four Germans, two Spaniards, one Russian, one Scot, seven Anglo-Indians, and three Americans. All of them were employed on well-defined terms.

Ranjit Singh never styled himself a monarch as such. For a long time he would not sit on a formal throne. He considered himself a leader of his people, a general selected by his community to fight for them. Says Vincent Smith, "The Punjab state was neither a traditional Indian territorial state and monarchy, nor merely a dictatorship of one community over another. There was an element of partnership with other communities. Ranjit did not claim the despotic sway of a traditional monarch over his own Sikhs. He was in some sense its elected chief and, like Augustus Caesar, he was careful never to push his pretensions too far. To the end, though taking the title of Maharaja, he claimed to be no more than a general of the Khalsa."

When Maharaja Ranjit Singh came to power it was the practice of the Sikh fraternity to get together at Akal Takht in Amritsar every time they had a major problem facing the community. It was called *Sarbat Khalsa*. They would debate the issue and a consensus decision would be made. Those decisions were binding on everyone and had religious sanction. The last such

Gurmatta passed by the brotherhood was in 1809 when Holkar sought refuge in the Punjab. He was being chased by Lord Lake of the East India Company.

The astute Ranjit Singh eventually found it convenient to replace *Sarbat Khalsa* by a council called "The Pillars of Kingdom." In this way "he formally effected a divorce between the spiritual and temporal affairs." Among the Pillars of Kingdom were Dhian Singh Dogra, a Hindu who was his Home Minister, and Fakir Azizuddin, a Muslim, who was his Foreign Minister. This was indeed a brave departure from a practice that everyone among the Sikh *misals* had come to respect.

After he assumed the title of Maharaja in a darbar in 1801, Ranjit Singh struck his own coins in a mint in Lahore. One of the coins had the following Persian couplet engraved on it:

Deg-o-teg-o-fateh-o-nusrat bedarang
Yaft az Nanak Guru Gobind Singh.

The words were both in Persian and Gurmukhi scripts. It is said that the Maharaja also issued coins called *Moranshahi Sikka* in honor of Moran, a Muslim courtesan, whom he had taken as a queen. The Sikhs never excused him for it. He was heavily fined but the coin remained in currency. Some people believe that *Moranshahi Sikka* was Maharaja Ranjit Singh's tribute to the womanhood of the Punjab since, rather than the image of Moran, his most favorite queen, he had *Arsi*—a thumb-mirror—carved on one side of the coin. The thumb-mirror was popular with society women in the Punjab in those days.

Although Maharaja Ranjit Singh was every inch a Punjabi, who would prostrate before the *Holy Granth* written in Gurmukhi script every morning, he did not have Punjabi as the state language. Persian continued to be the language of the court. He even encouraged his princes to learn foreign languages like English. He had some foreign works translated into Punjabi and is said to have granted a *jagir* to Shah Mohammed, a Punjabi poet of his time, who wrote an account of the Maharaja's expeditions with considerable devotion and skill. Along with propagation of Punjabi, he also gave endowments to Persian institutions like *Mian Wada* at Lahore.

There are a great many stories illustrating how Maharaja Ranjit Singh gave equal respect to all religions. The following is told by Fakir Syed Waheeduddin, a progeny of Fakir Azizuddin, Foreign Minister of Maharaja Ranjit Singh:

> On occasion the Maharaja and the Fakir were out walking on the outskirts of Lahore, when they met a bullock-cart carrying what looked like a huge book. The Maharaja stopped the bullock-cart and asked the driver what he was carrying. "Maharaj," replied the driver, "I am a calligraphist and this book is a manuscript of the *Holy Quran,* which is my lifetime's work. I am on my way to Hyderabad to sell it to the Muslim King of that country. I hear he is a very pious and generous man." The Maharaja turned to Fakir Azizuddin and said, "This man seems to think that there is nobody this side of Hyderabad who is pious and generous enough to pay him a good price." Then he asked the calligraphist, "How much are you expecting, my good man?" The calligraphist named what would be a huge sum for a manuscript of the kind even today—ten thousand rupees. Before the Minister could intervene, the deal had been closed. "Fakirji," commanded the Maharaja, "please see to it that the man is paid ten thousand rupees from the state treasury." Soon after the manuscript had been acquired, the Maharaja asked Azizuddin to read out to him a passage from it. Azizuddin read out *Sura Yusuf* (Chapter on Joseph) and then translated it for the Maharaja's benefit. "But Fakirji," remarked Ranjit Singh, "the *Granth Sahib* says the same kind of thing. What is the difference?" "None, Your Highness," replied the Fakir, "the goal is the same, only the paths are different." The Maharaja rewarded Azizuddin for this apt remark by making a gift of the manuscript to him.

Another story concerns Sardar Hukam Singh Chimni, a noted

general and a favorite of the Maharaja, who arranged the assassination of a man named Said Khan due to some personal enmity. When the Maharaja came to know of it, he was wild. He sacked the Sardar from service and fined him one hundred and twenty-five thousand rupees. The amount was paid to the bereaved family. Because there was no capital punishment in Maharaja Ranjit Singh's *raj*, it could have hardly been worse. Capital punishment was not awarded even when an attempt was made on the Maharaja's person.

Maharaja Ranjit Singh ensured that the administration of justice was properly organized. There were proper courts presided over by competent judicial officers. There were special courts for Muslims who wished to be administered by *shariat* laws. The Maharaja revived the offices of *qazi* and *mufti,* prevalent during the Mughal period. He organized the revenue system of the state by appointing Bhawani Das, a high official, as chief of the Finance Department. Revenue collection in the Punjab was no longer the responsibility of an Amritsar banker. According to one estimate, at the time of his death, Maharaja Ranjit Singh's army, including the irregulars, totalled 123,800 (92,000 infantry, and 31,800 cavalry and artillery), which is almost equal in size to the entire Indian army's strength on the eve of World War II in 1939. The artillery consisted of 384 heavy guns and 400 light guns.

In regard to public offices, it was merit alone that counted with the Maharaja. The only other consideration was his concern to give due representation to the various communities within the *raj.* Key posts were manned by the best talent from the various communities and even talented foreigners were included. In his book, entitled *The Real Ranjit Singh,* published recently in Pakistan, Fakir Syed Waheeduddin states: "As regards Muslims in particular, the author's family archives contain lists of Muslim officers in the higher and middle echelons. Among the top-ranking Muslim officers, there were two ministers, one governor, and several district officers. There were forty-one high-ranking Muslim officers in the army, two of them generals, several of them colonels and the rest holding other important ranks. There were ninety-two

Muslims who were senior officers in the police, the judiciary, and the legal departments, and the supply and stores departments." The Maharaja had a galaxy of talent around him. Among the Sikhs were Sham Singh Attariwala, Hari Singh Nalwa and Sher Singh. The Muslims were represented by the three Fakir brothers— Azizuddin, Nuruddin, and Immamuddin—General Ghaus Khan and Ilahi Bakhsh. Among the Hindus were Dhian Singh, Gulab Singh, Khushal Singh, Ram Singh, and Misr Diwan Chand.

The main Sikh temple at Amritsar called *Harimandir Sahib* was destroyed by Ahmed Shah Abdali in 1761. Maharaja Ranjit Singh had the temple rebuilt. Its periphery was laid with marble stones especially acquired from Rajasthan, and the dome was gilded later when the Maharaja annexed Kashmir to his territory. The temple has since come to be known as the Golden Temple. The Maharaja also had a number of mosques erected from state funds. A mosque was built in Lahore and dedicated to Moran, the courtesan-queen of the Maharaja. Several important mosques were granted endowments in the form of *jagirs* so that they would be properly maintained. Similar endowments were made to Hindu temples.

The Maharaja visited Hindu and Muslim places of worship as devotedly as he visited the Sikh holy shrines. During his royal tours, he visited varied places of pilgrimage. These included Punja Sahib, the famous Hindu temples at Kangra and Jammu, the well of Puran Bhagat, the mausoleum of Data Ganj Baksh and the shrine of Mian Mir.

Maharaja Ranjit Singh's secularism was typical of the eighteenth century. It was conceived in a spirit of compromise and enlightened self-interest. It was in this spirit that the people of Lahore including Muslims, Hindus, and Sikhs invited him to occupy the town and relieve them from the tyranny of the ruling triumvirate. It was in this very spirit that he had complete faith in the three Fakir brothers whose successors have remained ardent admirers of the Maharaja until today. It was evident that Maharaja Ranjit Singh had endeared himself to all his subjects, from the way prayers were offered in gurdwaras, mosques, and temples when he was taken seriously ill, before he passed away on Thursday, the 27th of June, 1839.

7.
Sikhs in the Freedom Struggle

The role of the Sikhs in India's struggle for freedom has not been fully appreciated. They fought against British rule as few others did. Proportionately, the number of Sikhs who died in India's fight for freedom far outnumbers any other sector of Indian society. There was hardly an agitation in which they did not participate, whether it was the *Swadeshi* Movement or the *Khilafat*, Partition of Bengal, or Quit India. They offered themselves for arrest by the hundreds and thousands, underwent the severest persecution, and suffered untold privation.

The Sikhs were the last in the sub-continent to surrender to the British, and they were the first to raise arms against them. Their so-called communal agitations helped make British rule unsteady and contributed considerably to the freedom movement. When the Sikhs succeeded in their agitation for the control of Sikh gurdwaras and pilgrimage sites, wasn't it Mahatma Gandhi himself who applauded their efforts in a famous telegraph message, "The first decisive battle of Independence won. Congratulations."

The Jallianwala Bagh massacre took place next to the Golden Temple, and the largest number killed were Sikhs. Where else in the modern world would you find people lying on the rails with their wives and children and getting dismembered just to stop a train of freedom fighters who needed to be fed and provided with fresh water? Not many can claim the valor with which Sardar

Bhagat Singh offered himself at the altar of India's freedom. It is said that he kissed the noose before he was hanged.

It is evident that the agitations launched by the Sikhs were a training ground for the bigger fight for the country's freedom. One just needs to consider the fact that all the front-rank Sikh political leaders in the Indian National Congress, before and after Independence, had been the Akali activists. These included such notables as Kharak Singh, Mangal Singh, Gurmukh Singh 'Musafir', Pratap Singh Kairon, Swaran Singh, Hukam Singh, Baldev Singh, Buta Singh, Giani Zail Singh, and Gurdial Singh Dhillon. Not only this, but Sardul Singh 'Caveeshar', who finally succeeded Subhash Chandra Bose as the Chief of the Forward Block, and Sohan Singh 'Josh', the veteran communist leader, were also at one time active Akali workers.

Good or bad, it has never been possible for the Sikhs to separate politics from religion. Dictated by the exigencies of the situation, Maharaja Ranjit Singh blended politics and religion when he came into his own as the first Sikh ruler. Baldev Singh, Swaran Singh and Hukam Singh, the nominees of Master Tara Singh, Chief of the Akali Party, were alienated one after another from their mentor when they joined the Congress Government at the Center. Such are the imperatives of Indian politics. Whatever their differences with the Union Government, the Sikhs of the Punjab, whether farmers or soldiers, laborers or traders, acquitted themselves splendidly in the three wars fought with Pakistan after India became independent. They continue to offer themselves for recruitment in the Indian forces far beyond their numerical proportion.

They inherited a badly neglected, arid part of the Punjab at the time of Partition. They have turned it into the granary of India. Claiming the highest per-capita income, the Sikhs have made a considerable contribution to small-scale industry as well. With a rare spirit of enterprise and hard work, they have made a success of whatever field they have entered, and even as they have spread all over the length and breadth of India, and to every part of the world, the Punjab has remained their homeland. And this is how it should be.

The Sikhs were always in the mainstream of the national life. This tradition continues as they fill some of the highest offices in the land and avail themselves of the unlimited opportunities offered by a big country like India. They are involved in India's fight for social justice today as vigorously as they once plunged themselves into the struggle for freedom.

The story of the Sikhs' fight for freedom goes back to the nineteenth century; in 1863 a splinter sect of the community called Kukas organized themselves under Ram Singh (1816-1885). They were a para-military sect given training in the use of weapons. They propagated strict *Swadeshi,* wore home-spun *khadi* (cotton), and led utterly austere lives. They boycotted British goods, and had nothing to do with British educational institutions or even British courts. They had their own postal arrangements to carry messages. Inevitably they clashed with the government and a large number of them were tied to barrels of guns and blown off or cut to pieces. Their leader, Ram Singh, with eleven of his close followers, was banished to Burma. He is said to have died in exile in 1885 pining for his motherland.

The next landmark in the Sikh struggle for freedom was the agitation launched against the Punjab Colonization Act, 1907, under which the Government sought to enhance land revenue and water charges in areas irrigated by the canal. There was widespread agrarian unrest, and bloodshed occurred in such important towns as Lahore and Rawalpindi. It was during this agitation that one Banke Dyal wrote the famous Punjabi song—*Pagdi sambhal jatta, pagdi sambhal aue* (Mind your turban, O tiller of the land, mind your turban). It became a popular patriotic song with the freedom fighters and continues to be sung even today. Sardar Ajit Singh and Lala Lajpat Rai were prominent among the leaders of the movement. They were both expelled from the country and imprisoned in Mandalay in Burma. After their release Ajit Singh went to Canada and joined the Ghadar Party of which he became an outstanding leader in due course.

The Ghadar Party was started by Sohan Singh Bhakna under the inspiration of Lala Hardyal. They pledged to end British rule in

India through an armed revolution and set up a Republic of India guaranteeing liberty and equality to all its citizens. They set up their headquarters in San Francisco. They had a view to retaining the secular character of their organization and made it a point not to discuss religion in their meetings; it was considered strictly a personal affair. They also would not observe any restrictions in the matter of diet. Soon they were to be joined by Kartar Singh 'Sarabha', Dr. Mathura Singh and Jawand Singh, who were later hanged in India. The Party established its branches in a number of towns in America, Canada, Shanghai, Hong Kong, the Philippines, Thailand, and Panama. They also provided training in arms for a select group of their members.

The activities of the Ghadar Party received a great stimulus by what has come to be known as the *Kamagata Maru* episode. It inspired the Ghadarites and steeled their hearts against the *ferringhi*. They were determined to throw off the foreign yoke and prepared themselves to make any sacrifice for this cause.

The *Kamagata Maru* was the name of a Japanese ship engaged by Baba Gurdit Singh for transporting Indian emigrants to Canada. Because there was widespread unemployment at home, more and more enterprising Punjabis sought to go abroad. And as Canada was a member of the Commonwealth, Indians were entitled to have free access to the country. However, with the support of the British Government, Canada passed an act presenting entry of Asians. This was primarily directed against the Indians since Canada continued to allow Chinese and Japanese to immigrate in large numbers.

The Sikhs would not have it. Accordingly, the *Kamagata Maru* with 376 passengers on board arrived at Vancouver on 22 May 1914. They were not permitted to disembark onto Canadian soil. The ship was stranded on the high seas. The passengers had no medicines. They even fell short of water. But the Canadian authorities would not relent. There was a skirmish with the local police, and it is alleged that gun fire was exchanged. The Government of Canada was not even willing to allow provisions for the return journey. This enraged the Indian community in Vancouver who threatened to set fire to the entire city. At this the Government appeared to see reason and the ship was allowed provisions for the return journey. The *Kamagata Maru* sailed back after two months. The returning passengers were provided arms *en route* at Yokohama, and the leadership of Baba Sohan Singh Bhakna and Baba Gurdit Singh turned each one of the passengers into a hard core revolutionary.

World War I having broken out in the meantime, the *Kamagata Maru* received a hostile reception when it landed in Calcutta. There was a train waiting to carry the passengers to the Punjab. This was not acceptable to the self-respecting Punjabis, who wished to remain in Calcutta and earn something, so that they didn't have to return home empty-handed. A confrontation ensued in which eighteen passengers were slaughtered. However, twenty-eight of them, including Baba Gurdit Singh, managed to escape. Baba Gurdit Singh remained underground for seven years until he surrendered himself to the police at Nankana Sahib, the birthplace of Guru Nanak.

The Ghadar party continued to produce revolutionaries for Indian politics. It is said, out of 8000 returnees during 1914-18, the Government of India interned 5000 and restricted the movements of another 2500. The Party had its sympathizers in the defense forces, though due to lack of discipline and leadership it could not take any precipitate action. Still, the Government was on their track, and suspects were arrested. Among 194 men taken into custody, 180 were Punjabis. Most of them were Sikhs and were charged with treason; as many as twelve were hanged. Some of them were imprisoned for life, others were deported, and the rest were given various prison terms.

Considering that the Indian National Congress session at Madras in 1914 had its main hall decorated with the portrait of the British King, and the Governor of the province was invited to grace the occasion with his presence, it was a great achievement of the Ghadar Party to do all that it did. Ultimately, its most significant contribution was to make the Britishers realize that they could no longer take India for granted. They must negotiate with the Indian people and hand over power to them, even if on a gradual basis.

When World War I was over the Punjab was in ferment. The forces being demobilized included 80,000 Sikh soldiers. By now Gandhi had assumed the national leadership. A great believer in the good faith of the white man, he was dismayed to find that the British Government had no desire to part with power. He, therefore, gave a call for *satyagraha*.

On the 13th of April, 1919, holy Baisakhi day, consecrated by Guru Gobind Singh with the baptism of the Sikhs, large crowds assembled at Jallianwala Bagh in Amritsar. They included men, women, and children. Brigadier General Edward Harry Dyer, who had arrived in the town two days earlier with his force, came to the scene, blocked the only exit, and started firing on the unarmed innocent people with machine-guns, "till all his ammunition was exhausted." The record says that 309 people were shot dead on the spot and many times that number were wounded. The Sikhs again suffered the largest number of casualties.

The people of the Punjab went wild with anger. They set post offices and other government buildings on fire, massacred any white men who came their way, removed fish plates from the railway lines, and cut telephone and telegraph wires. The entire Punjab was aflame. The government declared martial law and retaliatory measure were carried out all over the province.

The Punjab became the vortex of the political struggle. The Nobel Laureate, Rabindranath Tagore, relinquished his knighthood as a protest against the brutal Jallianwala Bagh massacre. The Indian National Congress held its annual session at Amritsar in December that same year. It was attended among others by Mahatma Gandhi, Motilal Nehru, Madan Mohan Malaviya, Jawaharlal Nehru, C. F. Andrews, C. R. Das, Dr. M. A. Ansari, the Ali brothers, and Hakim Ajmal Khan. Among the eminent Punjabi leaders who participated in it were Baba Kharak Singh, Lala Lajpat Rai, and Sardar Sardul Singh 'Caveeshar.'

The Sikhs now came to look upon Mahatma Gandhi and Jawaharlal Nehru as their national leaders and started seeking inspiration from them. They were in the vanguard of the political movement. The Sikh League held a meeting in Lahore presided over by Sardar Kharak Singh in 1920. The meeting was attended by Mahatma Gandhi.

It was about this time that the Sikhs launched what came to be know as the Akali Movement. Essentially aimed at taking charge of the Sikh shrines from the *mahants*—hereditary custodians—and bringing about reforms in the rituals and elaborate ceremonials, the movement went a long way in politicizing the Sikh masses and inculcating a passion for independence.

The Gurdwara Reform Movement was a gruelling struggle. The vested interests did not want to part with the charge of the Sikh shrines, some of which had considerable landed property attached to them, and were sources of substantial income. The Sikhs had to launch *morcha* (agitation) after *morcha*. At times the fight was directly with the government, while at other times the government appeared to back the hereditary custodians who were its proteges. In Delhi the government demolished a wall of the historical Gurdwara Rakab Ganj where the ninth Sikh Guru had been cremated. The Sikhs went wild. An agitation was launched. A *shahidi jatha* comprising Sikhs, Muslims, and Hindus, who were prepared to be martyred, left for Delhi under Sardul Singh 'Caveeshar'. The Government came to its senses and restored the wall of the holy shrine.

After the Jallianwala Bagh tragedy, the hereditary custodians of the Golden Temple invited Sir Michael O'Dwyer and honored him with a *saropa*. In the face of this outrage, how could the Sikh community allow the charge of the Gurdwara to remain in the hands of such inveterate toadies? Accordingly, another agitation was launched to take over the Golden Temple.

Mahant Narain Das of Nankana Sahib, the birthplace of Guru Nanak, was a debauch and a drunkard, who not surprisingly was pampered by the Britishers as well. A *jatha* of over 130 Sikhs who was visiting the Gurdwara were attacked with swords and spears by the *goondas* engaged by the Mahant and massacred. Their dead bodies were sprinkled with kerosene and burnt on the premises.

The leader of the *jatha*, Sardar Lachhman Singh, was tied to the trunk of a tree and lynched.

This tragic happening sent a wave of horror throughout the country. Mahatma Gandhi and the Ali brothers visited Nankana Sahib. The Government was alarmed. The charge of the Gurdwara was promptly handed over to a committee of Sikhs.

The Government, however, decided to appoint its own custodian for the Golden Temple. This was not acceptable to the Sikhs and the agitation continued. The agitators were sentenced to frightfully long terms of imprisonment. But there was no sign of the agitation abating anywhere. The Sikhs continued to protest and arrests numbered in hundreds and thousands.

At last the Government was brought to its knees and the keys of the Golden Temple were handed over to the Sikhs by the Deputy Commissioner of Amritsar at a huge congregation held in the town. This was described by Mahatma Gandhi as the first decisive victory in the battle for independence.

But what brought unique glory to the Sikhs was the *Guru Ka Bagh* agitation. A piece of land in Ajnala tehsil called *Guru Ka Bagh* (The Guru's Garden), which was no more than a barren tract with a wild growth of *kikar* trees, had been handed over to the Sikhs along with other shrines. However, Mahant Sunder Das changed his mind, and would not allow the Sikhs to enter the premises. The Sikhs used to fell trees in the arid tract to use as fuel for the community kitchen. The Mahant sought police assistance and the Sikhs entering the so-called *Bagh* were arrested for trespass. The first arrest took place on 8 August 1922. This was followed by a chain of Sikh *jathas* visiting *Guru Ka Bagh* one after another and offering *satyagraha*. The *jathas* came from all over the Punjab. There was an endless stream of them. It was intended to be a non-violent agitation. The Sikhs would go unarmed, singing hymns, with their hands folded and try to enter the land which belonged to their Guru. The police, who were tired of arresting them, adopted new tactics under a British Superintendent of Police named S.G.N. Beaty. They would beat the Sikhs mercilessly, pulling them by the hair, making indiscriminate lathi charges, breaking their bones, and inflicting grievous wounds on them. With the name of God on their lips, the *satyagrahis* would fall down unconscious but they would neither defend themselves nor retaliate. Many died, a large number of them had to be hospitalized, but there was no stopping the stream of *jathas*.

Though non-violence was advocated by Mahatma Gandhi, the Sikhs also had non-violence in their blood. Two of their Gurus— Guru Arjan and Guru Tegh Bahadur—had given their lives as non-violent crusaders. The way the Sikhs conducted this *satyagraha*, and the barbarities perpetrated on them, roused the anger of the entire nation. The Punjab was a flaming cauldron. Every district tried to outdo the other. A *jatha* came from far-off Dhani Pothoar with Giani Gurmukh Singh 'Musafir' (who became the Chief Minister of Punjab in Independent India) as one of the volunteers. A great many books were written about this unprecedented persecution and the valor of the non-violent *satyagrahis*.

It surprised Mahatma Gandhi, the apostle of non-violence, the most. He was amazed to find vindication of his technique of political warfare coming from the most unexpected quarters, the brave people of the Punjab. Several national leaders both Hindus and Muslims came to the Punjab to see with their own eyes the way the *satyagraha* was being conducted.

Pandit Madan Mohan Malaviya, a staunch Hindu who was at one time President of the Indian National Congress, witnessed the manner in which the disciplined soldiers of the Sikh community suffered barbaric treatment for this cause dear to their heart. He was moved to say, "I cannot resist asking every Hindu home to have at least one male child initiated into the fold of the Khalsa. What I see here before my eyes is nothing short of a miracle in our whole history."

C. F. Andrews, a Christian missionary and an associate of Mahatma Gandhi, also visited the Punjab during the *satyagraha*. This is what he reported:

"There were four Akali Sikhs with black turbans facing a bank of about a dozen policemen, including two English officers. Their hands were placed together in prayer. Then an Englishman without provocation lunged forward the head of his *lathi*, bound with brass, and struck the Sikh at the collar bone with great force. He fell to the ground, rolled over and slowly got up once more to face the same punishment till he was laid prostrate by repeated blows. Others were knocked out more quickly. It was brutal in the extreme. I saw with my own eyes one of those policemen kick in the stomach a Sikh who stood helplessly before him. I wanted to cry and rush forward. But then I saw a police sepoy stamping with his foot an Akali Sikh hurled to the ground and lying prostrate.... The brutality and the inhumanity of the whole scene was indescribably increased by the fact that the men who were hit were praying to God and had taken a vow (at the Golden Temple) to remain silent and peaceful in word and deed. I saw no act or look of defiance. It was a true martyrdom, a true act of faith. I reminded me of the shadow of the cross."

There were ever so many similar *morchas*. *Guru Ka Bagh* was followed by what has come to be known as the *Jaito Morcha*. Jawaharlal Nehru also joined hands with the agitating Sikhs here and courted arrest along with a number of prominent national leaders. Nehru made the following observation on the occasion:

"I rejoice that I am being tried for a cause which the Sikhs have made their own. I was in jail when *Guru Ka Bagh* struggle was gallantly fought and won by the Sikhs. I marvelled at the courage and sacrifice of the Akalis and wished that I could be given an opportunity of showing my deep admiration of them by some form of service. That opportunity has now been given to me and I earnestly hope that I shall prove worthy of their high tradition and fine courage. Sat Sri Akal."

Jawaharlal Nehru
25 September 1923

The Sikhs of the Punjab never allowed the white rulers any

respite. They kept them engaged with one *morcha* after another. And these agitations produced a galaxy of eminent freedom fighters who earned great names in the national struggle for India's Independence. Some of them are: Baba Kharak Singh, Master Tara Singh, Pratap Singh Kairon, Giani Gurmukh Singh 'Musafir', Sohan Singh 'Josh', Sardar Sardul Singh 'Caveeshar', Giani Zail Singh, Sardar Hukam Singh, Sardar Gurdial Singh Dhillon, and Darshan Singh Pheruman.

While the Shiromani Gurdwara Prabandhak Committee set up to take charge and look after the Sikh Gurdwaras accepted the cult of non-violence, there were certain elements among the Sikhs who organized themselves as underground terrorists. Among them the Babbar Akalis were perhaps the most virulent. Their members were drawn from the Ghadar Party and soldiers on leave. They issued a cyclostyled bulletin called *Babbar Akali Doaba.* For a while they became a terror for the adminstration in Jullundur Doab. They were led by Havildar Major Kishan Singh Bedang and Master Mota Singh. But eventually they were rounded up, and six of them including Kishan Singh Bedang were condemned to death and the rest were sentenced to various terms of imprisonment.

The Sikhs make fine soldiers. They are as loyal as they are valiant. They enlisted in large numbers both at the time of World War I and World War II. But after the wars were over and they discovered that the Britishers had no desire to part with power, they fought them tooth and nail. They were scandalized to find that the *ferringhi* would deny them the freedom for which he made them fight in far-off lands. They fought the war of India's Independence shoulder to shoulder with the rest of their countrymen, whether they were Hindus or Muslims, Beharis or Bengalis.

8.

Casting in Lot
With Secular India

The Sikhs were on the horns of a dilemma. The Muslim League was asking for Pakistan. The Sikhs were also an important minority, entitled to a separate identity, and a separate homeland. The British Government was willing to concede this, and it had indicated it unmistakably. Every time negotiations for the transfer of power took place, the Sikhs were included in the parlays in their own right, whether it was the Round Table Conferences or the Cripps or any other mission.

The Sikhs had another dilemma to resolve. On one hand, World War II was still raging. The brave Sikh soldiers were in great demand. There was unemployment at home. Recruitment to the forces would provide work and wage and more than anything else provide training, new skills, and awareness of modern society. The soldier returning home would help set up the small and medium-scale industries which were desperately needed. But, on the other hand, the Congress had decided not to cooperate with the war effort as long as the Government did not come to terms with it. So for the Sikhs on one hand, it was their enlightened self-interest, on the other the Quit India movement launched by Mahatma Gandhi. On the one hand, the Sikhs were offering themselves for recruitment to fight shoulder to shoulder with the British and on the other hand, they were courting arrests in the *satyagraha* launched by the Congress.

There was yet another predicament, a consideration that probably gnawed at the core of the Sikh sensibility. While the Muslims were close to the Sikhs in their faith, the Hindus were intertwined with them socially. They inter-married and they could dine together. This was seldom done with the Muslims.

And as regards historical perceptions, while the Muslims were unkind to the Sikhs, more particularly in the later part of Mughal rule, the Hindu rajas of the hill states were equally unkind in their harassment of Guru Gobind Singh and his followers. Even in modern times, while there were frequent clashes with the Muslims, the Sikhs had just as many grievances against the Hindus. It was, therefore, no easy task for them to make a choice.

Luckily, the leadership of the Sikh community at this crucial juncture was in the hands of Master Tara Singh, a man of sterling character, whose integrity was beyond question. A staunch Sikh, he had nothing but the interest of his people at heart. He was utterly truthful, and nothing could ever deflect him from a righteous path. Unafraid and outspoken, he had little use for so-called tact, diplomacy or political maneuvering. If the Sikhs ultimately decided to cast in their lot with secular India, the credit must go to Master Tara Singh alone. The Chief Khalsa Diwan or the Congressite Sikhs at the time carried little weight with the Sikh community; it was the Akali Dal that largely represented the Sikh masses, of which Master Tara Singh was the unquestioned leader. Like Mahatma Gandhi, it didn't matter if he held any party office or not. His modest house next to the Sikh Missionary College in Amritsar was the vortex of Sikh political activity, deliberations, and decision-making. Though self-opinionated, he never let his emotions have the better of him. A true Sikh, he always consulted his colleagues before arriving at a decision.

The first clear indication of the Sikh thinking regarding their choice is to be read in Master Tara Singh's letter to Sir Stafford Cripps of 31 March 1942 after his meeting with the Cripps Mission: "We have lost all hope of receiving any consideration. We shall, however, resist by all possible means separation of the Punjab from the all India Union." What had put off the Sikhs was the Cripps Mission postulating that immediately after the war was over, an elected body of Indians would be invited to frame a constitution with the provision that if any constituent of the Union wished to opt out of the Indian Union, it could do so. Evidently this was to accommodate Mr. Jinnah, who was insisting on an independent Pakistan.

The Sikhs had pinned their faith on the Congress leaders who they thought would not accept the creation of Pakistan. This was belied when C. Rajagopalachari came forward with his formula, which conceded the right of the Muslim majority provinces in the north-east and north-west to pull out if so established by a plebiscite. The worst part was that Rajaji claimed that his formula had the approval of Mahatma Gandhi. This enraged the Sikhs. A convention was held on 20 August 1944 in Amritsar in which Master Tara Singh, out of desperation, for the first time made the demand for an independent, sovereign Sikh State claiming that the Sikhs were a separate nation. However, it was rejected as an impossible demand at the same convention. Nevertheless, the convention appointed Master Tara Singh to organize the Sikh opposition to the division of the country or any part thereof.

Accordingly, the main issue on which the Sikhs fought the general elections of 1945-46 was opposition to the division of the country. They received a massive mandate. The communists among the Sikhs who supported the demand for Pakistan were routed in the elections.

The Sikhs' negotiations with the Cabinet Mission which visited India on the eve on Independence were highly frustrating. The negotiations were held under the overall leadership of Master Tara Singh, but the record shows that whoever met with the Mission, whether it was Giani Kartar Singh or Harnam Singh Advocate or Baldev Singh, all expressed somewhat different opinions. What they succeeded in convincing the Mission was that the Sikhs' demand for a separate State was not serious, but was only to counter the Muslim League's demand for Pakistan. And there was no denying it.

Accordingly, while reporting to the British Parliament, Sir

Stafford Cripps found the Sikh stand rather untenable: "What the Sikhs demand is some special treatment analogous to that given to the Muslims. The Sikhs, however, are a much smaller community, five and half million against 90 million Muslims and are not geographically situated, so that any area can be carved out in which they find themselves in a majority."

Exactly this position was stated by Master Tara Singh himself in his autobiography later: "We were aware of the fact that our case was weak for three reasons: 1) We asked for a Sovereign Sikh State if Pakistan were to be conceded. Our demand was, therefore, dismissed as counter argument, no one took us seriously; 2) The Hindus who appeared to support us did so to oppose Mr. Jinnah. In their heart of hearts, they did not subscribe to what we had asked for; 3) In the Punjab Legislative Assembly the Sikhs were divided with twenty-three Akalis and ten Congressites and then there were just two tehsils of Taran Taran and Moga, where the Sikhs were in a majority and those, too, were not contiguous."

Thus the Sikh demand for a separate Sikh State was never seriously put forward. And it was not considered seriously by any party. Eventually, when India came to be partitioned, what the Sikhs succeeded in was to partition the Punjab also, so that the Sikhs could cast in their lot with secular India and merge themselves in the mainstream of Indian society.

Even after Pakistan had been conceded in principle, the Sikhs had pinned their hope on the Boundary Commission since they somehow felt that their important shrines like Nanakana Sahib, the birthplace of Guru Nanak, and the canal-irrigated belt that they had developed with strenuous labor, would not be denied to them. They had a disappointment in store for them. With the announcement of the Radcliffe award, the Sikhs were equally divided between India and Pakistan. The Akali Dal under Master Tara Singh rejected the Award. However, they could not do much because their representative, S. Baldev Singh, who served in the Union Cabinet as Defense Minister, had already accepted it as a "settlement."

The Sikhs had to pay dearly for this settlement. Pakistan was determined to get rid of them. Communal riots took a frightful toll of Sikh life and property. They had to leave their hearths and homes and evacuate to East Punjab. Sir Francis Mudie, the governor of West Punjab, is said to have written to Mr. Jinnah, the Governor General of Pakistan, on 5 September 1947, "I am telling everyone that I don't care how the Sikhs get across the border. The great thing is to get rid of them as soon as possible. There is still no sign of three lakh Sikhs in Lyallpur moving, but in the end, they too will have to go."

While crusading for Pakistan, Feroze Khan Noon, a Muslim League leader, had announced, "If we find we have to fight Great Britain for placing us under a Central Hindu Raj, then the havoc which Muslims will play will put to shame what Chengiz Khan and Halaku did in the past." Exactly this is what was perpetrated on the helpless Sikhs and Hindus of West Punjab.

Their children were speared. Their womenfolk were abducted and raped. They were heartlessly slaughtered by hundreds and thousands. Their property was looted and their houses were set on fire. The police of the newly-created Pakistan, when not joining hands with the rioters, watched them from a distance. All this had its repercussions in East Punjab and the Sikhs and Hindus paid their neighbors in the same coin. The holocaust that followed has no parallel in Indian history—or in the history of the world.

It is estimated that not less than half a million human lives were lost in killings on both sides of the border. As many as five million Muslims were forced out of Pakistan and twice as many Hindus and Sikhs evacuated to India, the Sikhs concentrating mostly in East Punjab.

A herculean effort was required to rehabilitate them. But with the generous help of the Union Government and the indomitable spirit of the Sikh refugees from Pakistan, they were not only resettled, but they also converted what used to be an arid wasteland into a fertile region. When East Punjab came into being, it needed to import food, but today it is the virtual granary of India. The green revolution has brought prosperity to the farmers. Today, the Punjab claims the highest per-capita income in India.

They say every cloud has a silver lining. The Sikhs who were scattered all over the vast province came to be concentrated in what is known as Punjab, as a result of the partition. They have a State carved out on a linguistic basis. However small it may be, they are no longer discriminated against. They have an exclusive homeland of the Punjabi-speaking people. And as it is, the Sikhs enjoy majority status.

Crisis
in the Punjab

9.

Commitment
to Punjabi

According to the renowned Sikh Scholar, the late Principal
Teja Singh, Punjabi is the language that the people of the Punjab
have spoken from time immemorial. A living language keeps on
changing its complexion. During the course of history, this change
in complexion may result in the language being transformed
beyond recognition. Punjabi has undergone this metamorphosis
time and again and yet it remains Punjabi, the language to which
the people in this part of the country belong. Even today the
language spoken by the people living in Pothoar is different in
flavor from the one spoken in Malwa, as much as the language
spoken in Malwa is different in taste from that of Majha. It is said
that the dialects in India start changing about every 30 kilometers.
Like all other Indian languages, Punjabi, too, has a number of
dialects. They can be as diverse as Pahari, spoken in the north, and
Lehndi, prevalent in the south.

A language need not necessarily be conterminous with the
State boundaries despite the fact that in India we have tried to
reorganize the political map on a linguistic basis. The Punjab has
been particularly unfortunate in this exercise. The Punjabi-speaking people, already divided at the time of the partition of the
country into Pakistani Punjab and Indian Punjab, underwent
another bisection in our attempt to create the Punjabi Suba.

The Punjabi language has been plagued with yet another

malady. This pernicious ailment was inherited from its history. In the undivided Punjab before Independence, the Muslims majority was led to believe by the Britishers that Urdu and not Punjabi was their mother-tongue. Accordingly, they gave little importance to it. When they wrote in Punjabi, they employed the Persian script. Similarly, Hindus in the Punjab propagated the use of Hindi as prompted by the revivalist movements at the turn of the century. When they couldn't help writing in Punjabi, they opted for the Devanagari script. And finally the Sikhs, who remained unequivocally devoted to Punjabi as their mother-tongue, employed the Gurmukhi script that had been popularized by the Sikh Gurus.

The Sikhs have adhered to this Gurmukhi script because the *Holy Granth* was written in it. Yet this reliance on the Gurmukhi letters has created continual misunderstandings between the various communities over the years.

It has now been proven beyond any doubt that Gurmukhi script was prevalent in the Punjab long before the Sikh Gurus appeared on the scene. It was not Guru Angad, the second Sikh Guru, as is popularly believed, who invented the Gurmukhi script. He did propagate it. A great lover of children, he wanted Sikh children to be properly educated. He insisted on teaching them in their mother-tongue Punjabi, with Gurmukhi as the most suitable script for the purpose. In due course, the Gurmukhi script gained currency and recognition, so that when Guru Arjan Dev, the fifth Sikh Guru, decided to compile the *Holy Granth,* he opted in favor of this script.

The Gurmukhi script is drawn from Brahmi and Kharoshti scripts as is the Devanagari script. The two scripts share many common features. In the two alphabets, there are some similar sounds and some letters that look alike but have different sounds. Gurmukhi is a simple script, beautiful to look at, devised especially for the Punjabi language. It has continued to be modified from time to time, so that it eminently meets the demands of those who use the language today.

It is a truism that the Sikhs opted for the Gurmukhi script because it was prescribed by the Sikh Gurus. It is also a fact that the Gurmukhi script is best suited to the Punjabi language. It has been devised for it and during the course of years it has been modified to meet its changing needs.

The Sikhs' adherence to the Punjabi language is, perhaps, the most secular feature of their way of life. Accordingly, on the occasion of the creation of the Punjabi Suba, it was decided that the language of the people of the Punjab is Punjabi and its only script is Gurmukhi. It was a timely decision because the languages in India were then coming into their own. It put an end to all sorts of experiments that were in the offing.

It was only after Independence that the Muslims in the West Punjab belonging to Pakistan, realized that Punjabi and not Urdu was their mother-tongue. They learnt it the hard way. However, they continue to use the Persian script which makes their language drift further away from the language in use in our part of the Punjab. It is feared that if our Pakistani brothers do not see reason, before long their language will have an entirely alien character from the Punjabi prevalent in India.

While the Sikhs have adopted Punjabi with Gurmukhi script, many non-Sikhs have contributed to the development of the Punjabi language and literature. We have such notables as Dhani Ram 'Chatrik' the poet, Kirpa Sagar and I. C. Nanda, the playwrights, among the makers of modern Punjabi literature. They not only wrote in Punjabi, they also employed the Gurmukhi script. Their example is followed by a host of non-Sikh contemporaries who write with distinction in Punjabi. Most important among them are Devendra Satyarthi, the folklorist, Balwant Gargi, the dramatist, Dr. Roshan Lal Ahuja and Dr. Mohinder P. Kohli, literary critics, Harnam Das Sehrai, the novelist, Khalid Husain, the short story writer, Dr. V. N. Tiwari and Jaswant Rai, the poets. And, of course, there is Shiv Kumar Batalvi, who blazed a new trail in Punjabi and who recently passed away, mourned by millions of his admirers.

We have the *Holy Quran* and the *Ramayana* rendered into Punjabi. When Dhani Ram 'Chatrik' talks about Radha in his poetry, he is read no less avidly:

Udho, talk to me about Kanha
Don't you torture me any more
Hardly had the wounds started healing
When you came and opened them up again.

(Radha Sandesh)

Or when in our folksongs a Punjabi maiden longs for a spouse like Krishna, the cry is rooted in the soil of the Punjab.

Whom are you waiting for behind the *chandan* tree?
I wait for my father.

It's time, I should have a spouse, dear dad.
What type of spouse, dear daughter?
A spouse like the moon among the stars
And Krishna among the gods.

More than anything else, the Sikhs' commitment to the mother-tongue Punjabi is an abiding guarantee of their secularism. When the Punjabi Muslims flirted with Urdu and when the Punjabi Hindus turned their back on their mother-tongue, the Sikhs remained steadfast in their loyalty and devotion to Punjabi. This love for the mother-tongue is a chain which is going to bind us together, the Hindus, the Sikhs, and the Muslims of the Punjab.

Guru Nanak and the nine Sikh Gurus following him spoke to the people in their own idiom. They propagated the Punjabi language and the Gurmukhi script which they found admirably suited to their purposes. It would be a pity if this fact leads to any prejudices against the Punjabi language or the Gurmukhi script. The Punjabi language with Gurmukhi script is the common heritage of the people of the Punjab and it should serve as a cementing factor, binding the people into an eternal bond of understanding, good-neighborliness and brotherhood.

10.

A Crisis in Punjabi Identity

Punjab Needs a Composite Cultural Pattern

Every time I think of the Punjab, I see before my eyes a time-worn lady, a mother, with silken grey hair hovering over her radiant face, a glow in her soft eyes and haunting melodies murmured from her lips. She has long been on the road. Tired, she has taken up a staff, but her search continues as ever. She is Mother Punjab, looking for her identity. She is a feeble shadow of the real Punjab. She craves for the garden of which she is a faint fragrance. She longs to have a look at the rivers on whose banks she grew playing as a little child. She yearns for a glimpse of the mountains that gave her benign protection ever since she was born, and for the vast ocean that washed her feet with its tumultuous waters day and night.

As she walks along, she remembers the Punjab that was known as Sapt Sindhu, the land of seven rivers. The Punjab that folded in its arms Kabul and Kashmir, Ladakh and Sind. Then the Punjab of five rivers whose boundaries touched the Northwestern Frontier Province on one side and Delhi on the other. And then the Punjab that was split into two with a wedge drawn in blood in 1947, the Punjab belonging to Pakistan and the Punjab remaining an integral part of India. And then yet another Punjab that was vivisected further in Independent India. A Bodhi Tree trimmed in season and out of season. The Mother Punjab can hardly recognize what she now sees. Lost in memories she stares with a forlorn look at what remains of the Punjab.

Whatever may have happened to the Punjab, there is such a thing as Punjabi identity that must remain intact. And what is this Punjabi identity? According to Dr. H. D. Sankalia, the renowned anthropologist, "It is more or less established that at the end of the First Glacial Period and into the beginning of the Second Ice Age, Early Man entered the foothills of the Northwest Punjab, into the area traversed by the Soan, Haro and other rivers within the Indus-Jhelum Doab. Early man also spread into the area comprised by the Rawalpindi and Attock districts of the Punjab, and the Jammu and Kashmir States." Taking into account the findings of the Cambridge Expedition of 1935, Dr. Sankalia goes on to state, "The hand-axe industry is for the first time associated with the Soan flake and pebble industry at Chauntra, and here alone it reaches its acme, flowering into a fine late achulian type." Thus, a part of the Punjabi is the skill that Man developed on Punjab soil in Paleolithic, Neolithic, and Copper Ages and bequeathed to mankind. This was the skill to do things on one's own and not to look to others for succor. It was the craft of fine manipulation of one's fingers, the miracle of hard work, and the joy of invention. And it was an unswerving self-confidence, a pride in endeavor, and a capacity for strenuous labor.

Some 3,000 years before Christ, Mohenjodaro and Harrapa in the South of Punjab enjoyed a civilization as advanced as that of Egypt and Iraq. An eloquent testimonial to the level of development achieved by these cities is found in their carefully planned towns, their system of roads and streets, their extensive granaries and public baths, their ingenious drainage system, and their use of baked bricks, cement, and bitumen. One senses that these cities had an organized life, a dignified dress, and a concern for aesthetics in all aspects of life. Their houses were immaculately plastered, their crops were well-groomed, and their villages were neat and clean. Here was the Punjabi identity in the making.

It was on the soil of the Punjab that the *Vedas* came to be composed about 1,000 years before Christ. The musicality of their text and exuberance of their content lent liquid lyricism to Punjabi folksongs, lovelorn echoes to the Punjabi folktales and heroic overtones to the Punjabi ballads. And another part of the Punjabi identity is a love of music, a fondness for poetry and living life to sound like a symphony.

The Punjab forged its link with Ram Katha while founding Lahore and Kasur in the loving memory of Lav and Kush, the two sons of Sri Rama. The battle of *Mahabharata* was fought on the soil of the Punjab. It was on this soil that Lord Krishna gave his immortal message to Arjuna. While Sri Rama's union with his sons was a tender sequence of filial love, the *Mahabharata* stands for devotion to duty and unstinted sacrifice for a just cause. The Punjabi ethos came to represent respect for the truth, devotion to duty, a willingness to fight for justice, and faith in God.

Later in recorded history when Alexander the Great attacked India, the brave people of the Punjab snatched victory from the victorious even after having been vanquished. Alexander entered India storming everything that came his way and left as a chastened monarch making a friend of Porus. He changed his demeanor because he was convinced that even though the Punjabis had laid down their arms, in their hearts they had not surrendered. Victorious is he who doesn't accept defeat. The people of the Punjab have a tryst with destiny. They keep company with success, seldom encountering failure.

And this has been a way of life with them. When intruders came from the northwest, the Punjabis acted as the sword-arm of India. They bore the brunt of any attack and safeguarded the country's borders as best they could. The ballads of the Punjab sing of the brave deeds of its fighters. The soldier-lover figured in the Punjab folksongs frequently. The Punjabi youth became a symbol of heroism, sacrifice, and eternal alertness.

Be that as it may, the Punjabi did not lose faith in peace and harmony, brotherhood and amity. Born on its soil, Guru Nanak said, "There is no Hindu; there is no Musalman." All are human beings. This was his very first utterance after he was ordained. The other sufis and saints of Guru Nanak's time attempted a synthesis of Islam and Vedantist thought. It was marrying the Semitic creed with Aryan faith. Guru Nanak came to be known as the Guru of the Hindu and mentor of the Musalman. His people learned from him the values of good neighborliness and fraternity, to live and let live, and to forge friendship and cultivate lasting bonds.

What has been happening in the Punjab of late will put every right-thinking Punjabi to shame. People do have grievances but there are avenues in a democratic society to give vent to such grievances. The most unhappy soul in these current circumstances would be Guru Nanak himself, who strove for communal understanding and the brotherhood of man.

To my mind, we have been inevitably heading towards the situation existing in the Punjab today. Why we did not face this impasse earlier is a surprise. The seeds of communal distrust were sown a decade and a half ago when the Punjabi Suba in its present form came into being. It left every well-meaning Punjabi disenchanted, though Delhi, at a somewhat late date, conceded the concept of a Punjabi-speaking State in conformity with its commitment to reorganizing the provincial boundaries on the basis of language. However, it was left to a handful of narrow-minded politicians both at the Center and in the Punjab to work out the details. They played havoc with this task. The short-sighted Hindu saw to it that as much as possible was pared off the erstwhile State, so that the unilingual Punjab was left as diminutive as it could be. This same approach actually suited the parochial Sikh, who laughed in his sleeves. These machinations on the part of the bigoted Hindus were going to give a clear majority to the Sikhs in the new State. And this is what the diehard Sikh was looking for. It seems the people of the reorganized Punjab were driven to cast themselves into a narrow mold. It is no surprise that we are now suffering the consequences of these events.

This error of commission was followed by an equally grave error of omission. The successive governments in the Punjab, whether they were Congress, Akali or Janata, did precious little to foster healthy values or a composite cultural pattern in the State. Lost in a headlong race for banishing poverty by bettering performance in the fields and enhancing production in the factories, they neglected sensitive areas like art and culture. The result is that today the Punjab is utterly without any tradition of classical or light classical music. It has hardly anything better than Bhangra by way of dance. Its artists, whether Satish Gujral or Krishan Khanna, have become alien.

The creative writers are even worse off. The Punjabi writer who felt that the creation of the Punjabi Suba would open the flood-gates of opportunities was dismayed. The number of books published in Punjabi in 1980-81 was a bare 308 as against 1,046 in Bengali, 767 in Gujarati, 500 in Kannada, 1,044 in Malayalam, 1,361 in Marathi, and 1,135 in Tamil. It has become difficult to attract Punjabi authors like Rajinder Singh Bedi, Dr. Mulk Raj Anand, Khushwant Singh, Krishna Baldev Vaid, and Krishna Sobti to take to writing in Punjabi. Many eminent Punjabi authors are drifting away to Hindi and English. Punjabi theater is another name for vulgarity. A worthwhile production here and there is usually ignored.

After the green revolution, the Punjab is poised for an agro-industrial revolution. No one could stop the green revolution despite the water of the Punjab rivers being directed to neighboring states. The hardy Punjabi is going to usher in an agro-industrial revolution, even if he has to sweat without power and run his pumps with diesel oil month after month and year after year.

This new Punjabi is going to fritter away his energies in slogan-mongering and wasteful pursuits, if he is not given an opportunity to cultivate finer sensibility. He will indulge in vulgarity if he is not introduced to better pastimes. The new life makes a lonely modern man. The affluence, at times, can be frightfully destabilizing. It can kill the human in man, make him selfish and self-centered. We must guard against it. The time is here and now, if it is not already too late. All mischief is made in the mind of man and it is here that stable defenses against evil must be erected.

The media in the Punjab, therefore, have a grave responsibility. That they have miserably failed was proved recently when a senior journalist and a freedom fighter was slaughtered in a dastardly attack. Every phrase that is put to pen must be carefully weighed. We have all the freedom, but not the freedom to set our house on fire. In a recent survey by the Registrar of Newspapers, it was revealed that the Punjab has the largest number of periodicals including dailies, weeklies, and monthly journals. The responsibility of the press in the Punjab, therefore, becomes all the more grave.

Punjabi films continue to be as cheap as ever. The film in regional languages like Kannada and Malayalam, Bengali and Marathi has made long strides. The Punjabi film remains where it was. The Government must fill in the gaps wherever they occur. It must step in with appropriate support where a social or cultural need demands it.

The Radio and TV are the wings of the Government. They need to improve their image by better quality programs. Their propaganda broadcasts will carry conviction only if they improve their general performance. They must give their audiences aesthetically satisfying programs in order to cultivate their taste. It is hardly necessary to add that a lot more needs to be done in this respect.

And this brings me to creative writing, which is one of the most vital factors in keeping a people together. It has been the worst sufferer in the Punjab. The Punjabi writer is in a miserable plight. The people in the Punjab have yet to develop the reading habit. Since books don't sell and the Government has not purchased books in bulk for several years, publishing in Punjabi has virtually come to a grinding halt. The situation does not allow even a day's delay.

There should be a network of libraries in the State. It is the only way to foster the reading habit and it is also the only way to resuscitate our publishing industry in the present circumstances.

Those who read good books live in good company. Those who pursue fine arts have finer sensibilities and sharper perceptions. They have a wider vision and a larger heart. They have little time for narrow pursuits and parochial bickering.

Let the people of the Punjab read books so that they know why the greatest Sikh leader of our time, Master Tara Singh, chose to cast in the lot of his community with India when what is now called Khalistan could be had for the asking at the time of Independence.

What the people of the Punjab need is fostering the Punjabi identity. What is the Punjabi identity? It is love of the Punjab. It is love of the Punjabi language. It is love of the Punjabi way of life. A Punjabi is a good neighbor; "neighbors are born of the same parents," runs a Punjabi saying. A Punjabi is hard-working. "Work hard and share your earnings with others," said Guru Nanak. A Punjabi is ever ready to make any sacrifice for his land and his people, his tradition, and his heritage.

It bears repeating that commitment to the mother tongue is an imperative of the Punjabi identity. Love of the Punjabi language is the silken thread that should bind the people of the Punjab in eternal bonds. The need of the hour is to take pride in the Punjabi identity. Whether a Punjabi resides in the Punjab or Haryana, Himachal, or Delhi, Southall or Vancouver, he remains a Punjabi.

To be a Punjabi is to love the mother tongue and take pride in the Punjabi way of life. To be a Punjabi is to live in harmony and peace, and cultivate good-neighborliness and brotherhood. To be a Punjabi is to cherish one's heritage and love one's country. To be a Punjabi is to be progressive and lead a tension-free life. To be a Punjabi is to seek *sarbat ka bhala,* universal well-being. To be a Punjabi is to ensure that what others can do, a Punjabi does a shade better.

About the Author

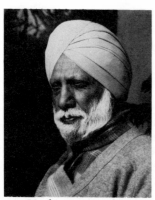

Kartar Singh (K. S.) Duggal, born in 1917, began writing while still a student. He is an author of repute in Punjabi, Urdu, Hindi, and English. His works have been translated into many other languages, and are used in literature classes in a large number of colleges and universities throughout the world. His published works include twenty-one collections of short stories, seven novels, seven plays, and two collections of poetry.

He has received numerous awards and prizes for his writing, including the Ghalib Award for Urdu Drama (1976), the Soviet Land Nehru Award (1981), the Fellowship of the Punjabi Sahitya Academy (1983), and the Bharatya Bhasha Parishad Award (1985).

His short story, "Come Back My Master" is included in the *Greatest Short Stories of the World.* He was recognized by both the Punjabi government (1962) and the Delhi Administration (1976) as a distinguished man-of-letters and awarded a "Robe of Honour." His collection of short stories, *Ik Chhit Chanan Di,* won the Sahita Academi award in 1965.

Mr. Duggal also served as Director of the All-India Radio from 1942 to 1966, as Director of the National Book Trust from 1966-1973, and was an Advisor (Information) to the Planning Commission from 1973 to 1976.

He has worked to encourage and promote literature and the arts throughout his life. He also served as a columnist for *The Indian Express, The Tribune,* and *The Indian Book Industry,* as a commentator on books, authors, radio, and television programs and the contemporary publishing scene in India.

Glossary

Amrit   Nectar

Ang   Limb

Ashtapadi   A poetic measure with eight couplets.

Badshahi Masjid   Royal mosque

Bandi Chhor   Liberator of the detained

Bani   Holy word

Baramah   A poetic form with a bearing on twelve months of the year

Bhakta   Devotee

Bhakti   Devotion

Chhand   Poetic measure

Degh   An oversize cooking vessel

Dharma   Faith

Doha   A poetic measure with two lines

Faqir   Muslim recluse

Fatwa   Verdict given by a Muslim divine

Gatha   A poetic form

Ghadar   Revolt

Goonda   Miscreant

Gurmata   Resolution of the Sikh religious body

Gursikh   Follower of the Guru

Harimandir   The abode of God. The name given to the Golden Temple at Amritsar

Jagir   Landed property

Jatha   Band

Kachha   Short pants

Kada   Bangle

Kafi   Poetic measure popularized by mystics in the Punjab

Kalma   The holy word

Kangha   Comb

Kesh   Hair

Khadi   Homespun cotton

Khanda   A double-edged weapon

Kikar   Acacia Arabica, a tree common throughout the Punjab

Kirpan   Dagger

Kripa   Goodwill

Langar   Common kitchen

Lathi   Stick

Manji   Seat

Maulvi   Teacher

Miri   Royalty

Misal   Band

Mohur   Gold coin

Mul Mantra   Basic postulate

Morcha   Agitation

Mufti   Magistrate

Mussali   A low-caste among the Indian Muslims

Pangat   Eating together

Panj Piare   The Five Beloveds who offered themselves to be martyred by Guru Gobind Singh

Patashas   Sugarcandy

Patwari   A village-level functionary who keeps land records

Piri   Renunciation

Qazi   Judge

Rabab   String instrument popular in the northwest of India

Raga   Musical form

Raja   Ruler

Sacha Padshah   True King

Sadhukari   Link language popularized by yogis in the north in the sixteenth century

Saje   Established

Sarbat Khalsa   Assembly of the Sikhs

Sardar   Leader

Saropa   Gift in recognition of merit

Sati   Immolation

Satnam   God is Truth

Seli Topi   A consecrated headgear

Shabad   Holy word

Shahidi Jatha   A band of volunteers pledged to be martyred

Shaikh   Muslim caste

Shakti   Power

Sharriat   Muslim law

Shikar   Hunting expedition

Siddhas   Hindu ascetics

Siharfi   Acrostic

Sikka   Coin

Sloka   Short poetic measure

Sufi   A mystic

Swadeshi   Indigenous

Swaiyya   A poetic form

Tegh   Sword

Var   Ballad

Walliallah   Beloved of God

Yunani   Greek—a system of medicine

Index

93

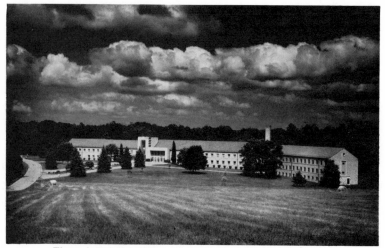

The main building of the national headquarters, Honesdale, Pa.

The Himalayan Institute

The Himalayan International Institute of Yoga Science and Philosophy of the U.S.A. is a nonprofit organization devoted to the scientific and spiritual progress of modern humanity. Founded in 1971 by Sri Swami Rama, the Institute combines Western and Eastern teachings and techniques to develop educational, therapeutic, and research programs for serving people in today's world. The goals of the Institute are to teach meditational techniques for the growth of individuals and their society, to make known the harmonious view of world religions and philosophies, and to undertake scientific research for the benefit of humankind.

This challenging task is met by people of all ages, all walks of life, and all faiths who attend and participate in the Institute courses and seminars. These programs, which are given on a continuing basis, are designed in order that one may discover for oneself how to live more creatively. In the words of Swami Rama, "By being aware of one's own potential and abilities, one can become a perfect citizen, help the nation, and serve humanity."

The Institute has branch centers and affiliates throughout the United States. The 422-acre campus of the national headquarters, located in the Pocono Mountains of northeastern Pennsylvania, serves as the coordination center for all the Institute activities, which include a wide variety of innovative programs in education, research, and therapy, combining Eastern and Western approaches to self-awareness and self-directed change.

SEMINARS, LECTURES, WORKSHOPS, and CLASSES are available throughout the year, providing intensive training and experience in such topics as Superconscious Meditation, hatha yoga, philosophy, psychology, and various aspects of personal growth and holistic health. The *Himalayan Institute Quarterly Guide to Classes and Other Offerings* is sent free of charge to everyone on the Institute's mailing list.

The RESIDENTIAL and SELF-TRANSFORMATION PROGRAMS provide training in the basic yoga disciplines—diet, ethical behavior, hatha yoga, and meditation. Students are also given guidance in a philosophy of living in a community environment.

The PROGRAM IN EASTERN STUDIES AND COMPARATIVE PSYCHOLOGY offers a unique and systematic synthesis of Western empirical sources and Eastern introspective science. Masters and Doctoral-level studies may be pursued through cross-registration with several accredited colleges and universities.

The five-day STRESS MANAGEMENT/PHYSICAL FITNESS PROGRAM offers practical and individualized training that can be used to control the stress response. This includes biofeedback, relaxation skills, exercise, diet, breathing techniques, and meditation.

A yearly INTERNATIONAL CONGRESS, sponsored by the Institute, is devoted to the scientific and spiritual progress of modern humanity. Through lectures, workshops, seminars, and practical demonstrations, it provides a forum for professionals and lay people to share their knowledge and research.

The ELEANOR N. DANA RESEARCH LABORATORY is the psychophysiological laboratory of the Institute, specializing in research on breathing, meditation, holistic therapies, and stress and relaxed states. The laboratory is fully equipped for exercise stress testing and psychophysiological measurements, including brain waves, patterns of respiration, heart rate changes, and muscle tension. The staff investigates Eastern teachings through studies based on Western experimental techniques.

Himalayan Institute Publications